yourself

indian head massage

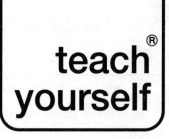

indian head massage
denise whichello brown

For over 60 years, more than
40 million people have learnt over
750 subjects the **teach yourself**
way, with impressive results.

be where you want to be
with **teach yourself**

Dedication
For my beloved Garry, Chloe and Tom

For UK order enquiries: please contact Bookpoint Ltd, 130 Milton Park, Abingdon, Oxon OX14 4SB. Telephone: +44 (0) 1235 827720. Fax: +44 (0) 1235 400454. Lines are open 09.00–18.00, Monday to Saturday, with a 24-hour message answering service. Details about our titles and how to order are available at www.teachyourself.co.uk

For USA order enquiries: please contact McGraw-Hill Customer Services, PO Box 545, Blacklick, OH 43004-0545, USA. Telephone: 1-800-722-4726. Fax: 1-614-755-5645.

For Canada order enquiries: please contact McGraw-Hill Ryerson Ltd, 300 Water St, Whitby, Ontario L1N 9B6, Canada. Telephone: 905 430 5000. Fax: 905 430 5020.

Long renowned as the authoritative source for self-guided learning – with more than 40 million copies sold worldwide – the **teach yourself** series includes over 300 titles in the fields of languages, crafts, hobbies, business, computing and education.

British Library Cataloguing in Publication Data: a catalogue record for this title is available from the British Library.

Library of Congress Catalog Card Number: on file.

First published in UK 2003 by Hodder Arnold, 338 Euston Road, London, NW1 3BH.

First published in US 2003 by Contemporary Books, a Division of the McGraw-Hill Companies, 1 Prudential Plaza, 130 East Randolph Street, Chicago, IL 60601 USA.

This edition published 2003.

The **teach yourself** name is a registered trade mark of Hodder Headline Ltd.

Copyright © 2003 Denise Whichello Brown

Typeset by SX Composing DTP, Rayleigh, Essex.
Printed in Great Britain for Hodder Arnold, a division of Hodder Headline, 338 Euston Road, London NW1 3BH, by Cox & Wyman Ltd, Reading, Berkshire.

Hodder Headline's policy is to use papers that are natural, renewable and recyclable products and made from wood grown in sustainable forests. The logging and manufacturing processes are expected to conform to the environmental regulations of the country of origin.

Impression number   10 9 8 7 6 5 4

Year   2009 2008 2007 2006 2005 2004

contents

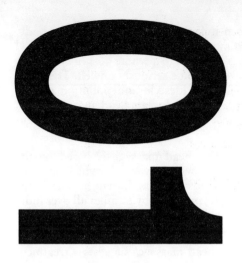

01

an explanation of Indian head massage

In this chapter you will learn:

- what Indian head massage is
- the physiological, psychological and spiritual benefits of Indian head massage
- the history of Indian head massage.

Indian head massage is a holistic therapy that balances body, mind and spirit, and promotes health and well-being. If we feel unbalanced, this 'dis-ease' can lead to a whole host of symptoms and diseases. We may even become seriously unwell. The stress of modern life, poor diet and lifestyle and pollution can all unbalance and block our energy. Indian head massage is an invaluable way to rebalance us, encourage healing and prevent diseases from occurring.

The traditional art of Indian head massage is based on the ancient system of medicine known as *Ayurveda*, which has been practised in India for thousands of years. Indian head massage has evolved from a technique, practised by families all over India as part of their everyday life, into a very comprehensive, popular and fast growing therapy carried out worldwide.

Although the term 'Indian head massage' suggests a treatment restricted to the head only, massage is also performed on the neck, shoulders, upper back and arms. Indian head massage is a very safe, simple, natural and gentle treatment usually performed with the receiver in a sitting position. It requires no special equipment and can be carried out through clothes. A complete Indian head massage treatment will only take about 30 minutes.

This book will enable you to master the Indian head massage techniques necessary to calm, uplift and revitalize your family and friends. What's more, it is incredibly rewarding – a head massage is as pleasurable to give as it is to receive.

What are the benefits?

Indian head massage offers a wide range of benefits for every system of the body – physiological, psychological and subtle/spiritual benefits.

Physiological benefits

Indian head massage helps to balance every system of the body.

Circulatory system

Indian head massage improves the blood supply to every part of the body. It distributes fresh blood carrying vital supplies of oxygen and nutrients to the cells, and takes away their waste products such as carbon dioxide. Oxygen and nutrients are carried to the tissues by the blood in the arteries and waste products are removed from the blood via the veins. As the tissues are nourished, healing is encouraged.

Indian head massage particularly improves the circulation to the brain, scalp, face, neck and shoulders. This increased supply of blood flow to these areas encourages alertness of mind and body, prevents muscle stiffness and will improve the condition of the skin and hair.

Indian head massage is also beneficial for cardiac problems because it can lower blood pressure and regulate and strengthen the heart.

Lymphatic system

Indian head massage boosts the efficiency of the lymphatic system. Any toxins, waste products and excess fluid that have accumulated in the tissues can be eliminated. Our body's defence mechanisms are stimulated, enabling us to fight off infections and recover more rapidly from illness. As our immunity to disease is strengthened, we become far less susceptible to coughs and colds, and other illnesses.

Muscular system

Indian head massage is an excellent therapy for relieving pain and stiffness from the muscles of the face, scalp, neck, upper back and shoulders. Muscles that are tense and contracted are not relaxed. The massage movements stretch and separate the muscle fibres so that muscles are able to relax as well as function to their fullest capacity. Tension headaches and aches and pains in the neck and shoulders may be reduced considerably as knots and nodules are broken down.

Waste products such as lactic acid that may accumulate particularly after exercise causing stiffness and muscle fatigue are removed more efficiently. Pain and stiffness in the muscles is relieved.

Skeletal system

Indian head massage eases stiffness in the joints increasing mobility in the neck and shoulder area. Any adhesions in the joints which are impairing flexibility may be broken down and the range of movement increased. Stiffness and pain arising from skeletal conditions such as arthritis are reduced providing ease of movement.

Hair

Indian head massage increases the circulation to the scalp, thus promoting hair growth. The hair becomes strong, shiny and healthy as blood flow is stimulated to the follicles bringing a good supply of nutrients and oxygen necessary for the growth of lustrous hair. The sebaceous glands which secrete sebum, the hair's natural moisturizer, are stimulated giving the hair a glossy sheen.

Skin

Indian head massage improves circulation to the skin, promoting a healthy and glowing complexion. The shedding of dead skin cells (desquamation) is encouraged so that fresh new cells are exposed giving the skin a healthier appearance.

The sebaceous and sweat glands are stimulated improving their function and ensuring that waste products are more efficiently eliminated through the pores. Sebum helps to keep the skin soft and supple, and the sweat glands unblock any clogged pores and remove toxins.

As with regular massage, the condition, colour, texture and tone of the face improves reducing the appearance of fine wrinkles, giving the face a much younger appearance.

Eyes

Indian head massage relaxes and soothes tense eye muscles. Eye strain is alleviated and the eyes may become bright and clearer.

Nose

Indian head massage is excellent for relieving nasal congestion and conditions such as sinusitis. The facial massage encourages mucous to be released and helps to improve our sense of smell.

Jaw

Indian head massage helps to alleviate jaw problems. As we clench our teeth and 'grin and bear it', this creates a great deal of tension in the jaw area which is easily dispelled via facial massage.

Psychological benefits

Stress and tension

Indian head massage is excellent for relieving stress and tension. A certain amount of 'positive' stress can be healthy, for instance, it can provide us with the motivation to complete a project or raise our performance when taking exams. However, we all have our own stress threshold and prolonged or high levels of stress result in exhaustion, both physical and mental. Minor problems now become major obstacles and health can become seriously affected.

The mind may become full of thoughts which go round and round in the head resulting in agitation and insomnia. Indian head massage can calm the mind and help to reduce sleeping problems. Some recipients fall asleep during a treatment and report sleeping much better and feeling more refreshed than ever before. Repressed feelings and tension can build up in the body. Feelings of hopelessness and despair and low self-esteem can collect and individuals become depressed and tearful. Desperation can even lead to aggressive behaviour. Indian head massage helps to release all of these emotional disturbances so that you feel calmer and able to cope with the pressures of everyday life.

The release of endorphins from the brain is stimulated, which counteracts the stress hormones and makes us feel good. The mood is elevated, anxiety and depression lifts and recipients feel uplifted and full of confidence.

Improved concentration

Indian head massage increases the supply of oxygen to the brain. This relieves mental fatigue and improves clarity of thought and concentration. Creativity and new ideas flow much more easily and productivity is increased.

Raised energy levels

Indian head massage increases our energy levels. Any energy that has become stagnant and blocked by tension is released and begins to flow freely. During a treatment a deep sense of peace and tranquillity is induced followed by an increase in energy levels. The mind and body is allowed to switch off and recharge. Afterwards individuals feel exhilarated and full of vitality.

Subtle/spiritual benefits

Indian head massage works on our subtle energy centres otherwise known as the chakras. These centres are unblocked, balanced and aligned at the end of a treatment allowing balance and harmony to be restored to body, mind and spirit.

Caution!

Indian head massage should never be used *instead* of orthodox medicine. It is complementary to orthodox medicine. Although a fully qualified, experienced Indian head massage therapist with a thorough grounding in anatomy and physiology may have the expertise to alleviate a wide range of health problems, the advice of a doctor should always be sought for persistent health problems.

A brief history

Massage is the oldest form of medicine known to humans and has been practised for thousands of years. As already mentioned, the ancient art of Indian head massage originates from the Indian system of medicine known as *Ayurveda*. This Sanskrit word can be translated as the 'science of life', 'knowledge of life' or the 'science of longevity'. The Ayurvedic approach to health is the balance of body, mind and spirit, and the promotion of long life. This system recommends the use of massage together with diet, herbs, cleansing, yoga, meditation and exercise.

Massage has always played an essential role in family life in India. It is an integral part of the daily routine and is highly recommended for both males and females throughout all the stages of life.

- **Babies.** It is customary for Indian babies to be massaged every day from birth until the age of three. This encourages the bonding process, keeps baby healthy and happy and helps to create a secure family environment.
- **Children (3–6).** At the age of three until the age of six Indian children are massaged two or three times a week. Some mothers still continue to massage their children every day.
- **Children (7+).** When the children are seven they will begin to learn the ancient techniques of massage. By experiencing massage and by observing other members of the family carrying out a massage treatment they will begin to grasp the techniques. Gradually they begin to perform massage on other family members.
- **Prior to a wedding.** It is customary for both the bride and groom to receive a massage before the wedding ceremony. This helps to relax the couple and promotes beauty, health and stamina as well as fertility.

- **Pregnancy**. Expectant mothers are massaged throughout pregnancy and for a minimum of 40 days after the birth of the baby.
- **Later life**. Massage continues to be part of family life right into old age. A grandparent will be given a massage by another member of the family perhaps by a grandchild.

Thus, massage plays an important role in family life. Indian head massage was originally developed by women as part of their daily grooming routine. Massage skills were passed on from mother to daughter from generation to generation. The oils such as sesame, almond and coconut that they massaged (and still do) into their scalps assured a healthy scalp and beautiful, long, lustrous, glossy hair.

Indian barbers incorporate massage into their treatment. A visit to the barber will always involve *champi* – the Western word 'shampoo' is derived from this word which means 'having your head massaged'. Barbers perform a stimulating, invigorating head massage that leaves their clients revitalized and alert. A barber will pass on his particular techniques to his son. Everyone has his or her own individual techniques.

Massage is not only practised in the home and at the barber's but is available on every street corner. On every beach you will be able to receive an Indian head massage.

Indian head massage has only recently been introduced to the West but has become enormously popular. It is one of the fastest growing therapies and is taught in many colleges all over the world. Indian head massage is an extremely popular therapy in the workplace since there is no need to disrobe, no equipment is required, the treatment is quick and easy to perform, and it is very effective.

02

all about the head and face

In this chapter you will learn:

- the bones of the skull
- the bones of the neck and shoulder region
- the muscles of the head and face
- oriental diagnosis of the head and face.

The structure of the skull

It is important to have some knowledge of the bones and muscles of the skull, neck and shoulders before giving a massage. This will increase your awareness of which areas should be massaged and which should be avoided, and thus optimum benefit can be derived.

The skull, which provides protection for the brain, is made up of 22 bones and is composed of two parts:

1 the cranium (eight bones)
2 the face (14 bones)

The cranium

The eight cranial bones are as follows:

• frontal bone
• parietal bones (two)
• temporal bones (two)
• occipital bone
• sphenoid bone
• ethmoid bone.

Frontal bone

The frontal bone forms the forehead and the anterior part of the top of the cranium. It also forms the roofs of the orbits (eye sockets). It contains the frontal sinuses and joins with the two parietal bones by the coronal suture.

Parietal bones

The two parietal bones form a large portion of the sides and roof of the cranium. They make joints with several bones: the lambdoidal suture with the occipital bone; the squamous suture with the temporal and sphenoid bones; the coronal suture with the frontal bone.

Temporal bones

The two temporal bones form the lower sides of the cranium. The term 'tempora' means temples. The bones house the structures of the middle and inner ear.

Occipital bone

The occipital bone forms the lower posterior (back) part of the skull. It makes joints with three other cranial bones – parietal, temporal and sphenoid. The occipital bone has a large hole called the foramen magnum through which the upper part of the spinal cord passes.

Sphenoid bone

The sphenoid bone is located at the middle part of the base of the skull. The word 'spheno' means wedge. This bone is referred to as the keystone of the cranial floor. It articulates with all the other cranial bones and also forms part of the eye socket. The sphenoid bone resembles a bat with its wings outstretched and its legs extended down and back.

Ethmoid bone

The light, spongy ethmoid bone is found between the orbits. It is anterior to the sphenoid yet posterior to the nasal bones.

The face

The 14 facial bones are as follows:

- nasal bones (two)
- maxillae (two)
- zygomatic bones (two)
- mandible
- lacrimal bones (two)
- palatine bones (two)
- inferior nasal conchae (two)
- vomer.

Nasal bones

The two small oblong nasal bones form the upper part of the bridge of the nose. The lower part of the nose is made up of cartilage.

Maxillae

The two maxillae unite to form the upper jaw. They serve as the keystone of the architecture of the face and articulate with every bone of the face except the mandible (lower jaw bone). The maxillae form most of the hard palate (roof) of the mouth, part of the floor of the orbits and part of the nasal cavities. Each maxillary bone contains a maxillary sinus.

Zygomatic bones (malars)

The two zygomatic bones (malars) shape the cheekbones primarily but also form part of the orbits. They articulate with the frontal, temporal, sphenoid and maxillary bones.

Mandible

The mandible is the largest and strongest bone of the face and forms the lower jaw. It articulates with the temporal bones.

Lacrimal bones

The two lacrimal bones form the medial (inner) wall of the orbit (eye socket). They are the smallest bones in the face, almost paper thin and about the size and shape of a fingernail. The lacrimal (tear) bones are named because they contain grooves for the nasolacrimal duct (tear duct).

Palatine bones

The two palatine bones unite together in the midline like two Ls facing each other. They form the posterior part of the roof of the mouth (hence palate), the floor and sidewalls of the nose and a small portion of the floors of the orbits.

Inferior nasal conchae (turbinates)

The two inferior nasal conchae are scroll-like in shape and form the outer walls of the nose. (The superior and middle conchae are part of the ethmoid bone.)

Vomer

The triangular vomer bone forms part of the nasal septum (the ethmoid bone and septal cartilage complete the septum).

If the vomer is deviated (pushed to one side), the nasal chambers are of unequal size and therefore nasal congestion and even chronic sinusitis is likely.

Bones of the neck and shoulder region

The neck

The neck is composed of seven cervical vertebrae. The first cervical vertebra is also known as the *atlas*. The atlas supports the head. The second cervical vertebra, known as the *axis*, allows the head to rotate.

The shoulders

The shoulder girdle, which allows movement of the shoulders, is composed of the following bones:

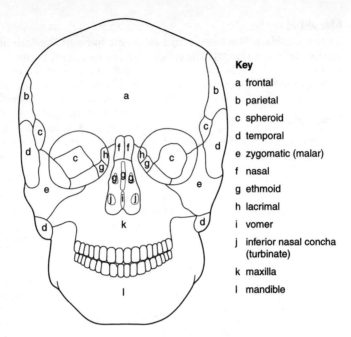

Key

a frontal
b parietal
c spheroid
d temporal
e zygomatic (malar)
f nasal
g ethmoid
h lacrimal
i vomer
j inferior nasal concha (turbinate)
k maxilla
l mandible

figure 1 skull viewed from front

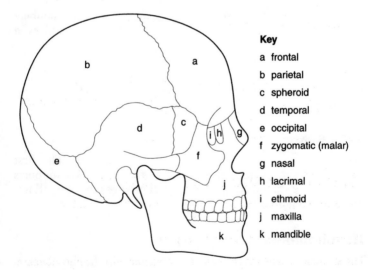

Key

a frontal
b parietal
c spheroid
d temporal
e occipital
f zygomatic (malar)
g nasal
h lacrimal
i ethmoid
j maxilla
k mandible

figure 2 skull viewed from side

- **Two clavicles.** The clavicles (collar bones) are long, slender bones which articulate with the scapulae (shoulder blades) and the sternum (breastbone).
- **Two scapulae.** The two triangular-shaped shoulder blades are found in the upper back – one each side of the spine.

The upper arms

The humerus is the bone located in each upper arm. The head of the humerus articulates with the scapula in a ball and socket joint and allows for a variety of movements.

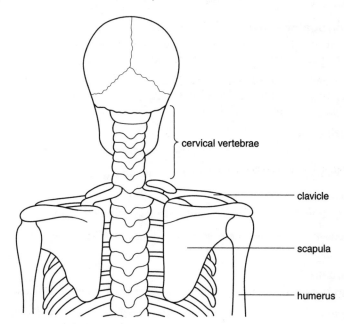

figure 3 the bones of the neck and shoulder area

Muscles of the head and face

The following are the main muscles of the head and face.

Muscles of facial expression

These muscles are responsible for a remarkable range of facial expressions.

Occipitofrontalis

Position: The occipitalis and the frontalis are collectively known as the occipitofrontalis. This muscle is also known as the epicranius. The occipitalis (epicranial frontal belly) is a muscle sheath extending over the back of the skull (the occipital bone). The frontalis is a sheath of muscle over the front of the skull (the frontal and parietal bones). Together they cover the skull rather like a cap.

Action: Occipitalis draws the scalp backwards; frontalis moves the scalp forwards (wrinkles the forehead horizontally) and raises the eyebrows.

Corrugator supercillii

Position: The corrugator muscles are small muscles located between the frontal bone and the skin of the eyebrows.

Action: They draw the eyebrows down and towards each other, i.e. they wrinkle the forehead vertically to produce a frown (*corrugo* means to wrinkle).

Procerus

Position: The small procerus muscles are found on the nasal bones.

Action: They wrinkle the nose to create an expression of disgust!

Orbicularis oculi

Position: The orbicularis oculi muscles encircle the eyes.

Action: They close the eyes. If you wink or blink these muscles are used.

Nasalis

Position: The nasalis muscles cross over the bridge of the nose.

Action: They dilate (open up) the nostrils and are used when flaring the nostrils!

Levator labii superioris

Position: These are thin bands of muscles running from under the eye to the mouth.

Action: They raise the upper lip producing a cheerful expression.

Zygomaticus (minor and major)

Position: This thin muscle pair extends diagonally from the zygomatic bones to the angle of the mouth (major) and to the upper lip (minor). They are superficial to the masseter muscles.

Action: They draw the angle of the mouth upward and backward as in laughing.

Levator anguli oris

Position: These thin bands of muscle run from the maxilla to the corner of the mouth. They lie below the levator labii superioris.

Action: They raise the corner of the mouth producing a cheerful expression.

Buccinator

Position: These are the major muscles of the cheek lying deep to the masseter muscles (*bucc* means cheek).

Action: They are used for whistling and also blowing as when playing a trumpet. The buccinator muscles also draw the cheeks in towards the teeth as when chewing.

Risorius

Position: The risorius muscles run towards the corners of the mouth.

Action: They retract the angle of the mouth as when grinning (*risor* means laughter).

Orbicularis oris

Position: The orbicularis oris encircles the mouth.

Action: It closes and protrudes the lips as in kissing.

Depressor anguli oris (triangularis)

Position: These muscles extend from the mandible to the corners of the mouth.

Action: They pull down the corners of the mouth as when frowning.

Depressor labii inferioris

Position: These muscles are located between the mandible (mid-chin) and skin of the lower lip.

Action: They draw the lower lip downwards to create a sulky expression.

Mentalis

Position: The mentalis muscles form a V-shape over the centre of the chin.

Action: They raise and protrude the lower lip and also wrinkle the skin of the chin.

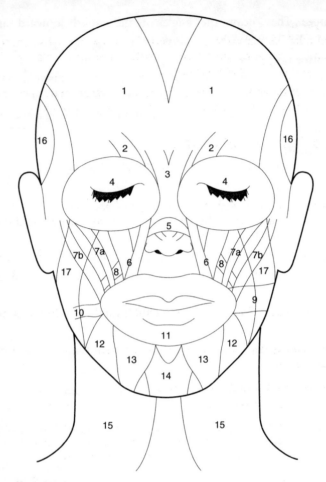

Key

1 frontalis part of the epicranius
2 corrugator supercilii
3 procerus
4 orbicularis oculi
5 nasalis
6 levator labii superioris
7a zygomaticus minor
7b zygomaticus major
8 levator anguli oris

9 buccinator
10 risorius
11 orbicularis oris
12 depressor anguli oris (triangularis)
13 depressor labii inferious
14 mentalis
15 platysma
16 temporalis
17 masseter

figure 4 muscles of facial expression and mastication

Platysma
Position: The platysma is a superficial broad sheet-like muscle extending from the upper fourth of the chest up the sides of the neck to the chin, jaw and mandible.

Action: It depresses the lower lip and also draws up the skin of the chest. The platysma muscle is used when yawning.

Muscles of mastication

The following muscles are responsible for chewing.

Temporalis
Position: The fan-shaped temporalis muscles are at the side of the head and extend from the temporal bone in front and above the ear down to the lower jaw.

Action: They close the lower jaw, clench the teeth and help with the chewing action.

Masseter
Position: The masseter muscles extend from the cheekbone to the mandible.

Action: They close the lower jaw and clench the teeth (*maseter* means chewer).

Pterygoids (medial and lateral)
Position: The pterygoids are deep muscles which act on the jaw.

Action: The medial pterygoid closes the lower jaw and clenches the teeth. The lateral pterygoid opens the jaw, protrudes the mandible and moves the mandible from side to side.

If you would like more details of muscles of the neck, shoulders and arms, you can refer to *Teach Yourself Massage*.

Oriental diagnosis

The principles of the fascinating art of oriental diagnosis were developed and preserved in Japan, China, Korea and India for many centuries among religious, cultural and philosophical traditions. The basic principles of oriental diagnosis can be found in such classics texts as *The Yellow Emperor's Classic of Internal Medicine*, *The Book of Changes* and *Karaka Samhita*. Oriental diagnosis not only reveals the presence of many existing disorders but can also detect potential problems before they arise. Thus, it is possible to prevent illnesses from occurring. As you will discover, the face and head reveal a great deal about the physical and mental condition of an individual.

The face

Each organ of the body is reflected on a specific area of the face. This is a similar idea to reflexology where all the structures and organs can be seen in miniature on the hands and the feet (see *Teach Yourself Hand Reflexology* for more information). Thus our faces are a mirror of our health.

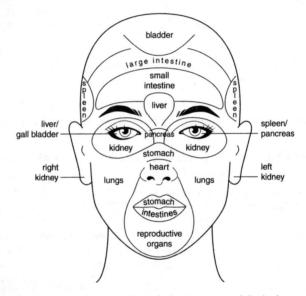

figure 5 areas of the face and their relation to organs of the body

The forehead

Upper part

The upper part of the forehead represents the condition of the bladder.

Middle part

The middle part of the forehead reveals the large intestine.

Lower part
The part of the forehead above the eyebrows is related to the small intestine.

Temples
The temples reflect the condition of the spleen.

Between the eyebrows
The liver is represented in the area between the eyebrows.

The nose

Upper part
The upper part of the nose is related to the pancreas.

Middle part
The stomach is represented on the middle part of the nose.

Tip
The tip of the nose reflects the heart and the nostrils mirror the bronchi.

The eyes

The area of the eyes reveals the condition of the kidneys and the reproductive organs (ovaries in a woman, testes in a man). In addition, the right eye reflects the liver and gall bladder areas whereas the left eye represents the spleen and pancreas.

The ears

The ears are related to the kidneys – the right ear to the right kidney, the left ear to the left kidney.

The cheeks

The cheeks are related to the lungs.

The mouth

The lips in general show the condition of the digestive system.

Upper lips
These are related to the stomach.

Lower lips
These reveal the intestines.

Corners
The corners of the lips represent the duodenum.

The chin
The chin and the area around the mouth represent the reproductive organs.

The head

Centre of the top of the head
This area reveals the condition of the heart and the small intestine.

Around the central part
The digestive system is reflected in the area surrounding the centre of the top of the head.

Back of the head
The back of the head mirrors the liver, spleen and pancreas.

Sides of the head
The sides of the head represent the lungs.

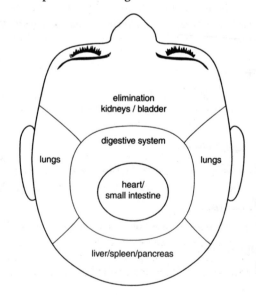

figure 6 the top of the head

Front of the head

The frontal part is connected with the organs of elimination and in particular the kidneys and bladder.

Now that you have a general picture, let us examine some of these areas in more detail.

The forehead

In general a clear forehead indicates excellent physical and mental health.

Upper forehead

The upper region of the forehead is related to the circulatory and the excretory systems. If this area is well developed, it indicates a strong heart and healthy kidneys and bladder. A well-balanced upper forehead also indicates an understanding of the spiritual world.

If there are pimples, this is indicative of the over-consumption of various foods – white pimples from fats and oils, red pimples from sugar, yellow pimples from animal fats and dark pimples from proteins and fats together.

A red upper forehead appears if the circulatory functions are overworked, causing a fast pulse. Overactive excretory functions result in frequent urination and diarrhoea. White patches may appear if too many dairy products are consumed, resulting in high cholesterol and accumulation of mucous. Excessive sugar shows up as dark colour and patches, with the possibility of kidney stones and frequent bladder infections.

Middle forehead

This area represents the nervous system. Good development of this region shows a sound intellect.

A white colour in the middle forehead usually indicates sluggish mental functions whereas redness shows nervousness and oversensitivity. Pimples, white, yellow or dark patches may also be evident due to the reasons given in the upper forehead section.

Lower forehead

If the lower region of the forehead is well developed, the digestive and respiratory systems are strong and the physical and mental energies are good. Vertical wrinkles in between the eyebrows indicate a hardening and stagnation of the liver. They also show a tendency towards anger and temper tantrums. Redness across the lower forehead is a warning that inflammation may be developing in the digestive or respiratory organs. A darkening of this area shows a slow metabolism and constipation, or breathing problems are possible. Patches and pimples may also be present.

Temples

The temples relate not only to the spleen but also to the pancreas, liver and gall bladder. If this area is greenish this indicates an underactive gall bladder or an overactive spleen. A dark colour appearing in this region shows underactivity in the spleen and liver and the possibility of malfunction of the pancreas. Pimples and patches may also be present.

The nose

The nose is a mirror of the nervous and circulatory systems as well as some aspects of the digestive system. A well-formed nose shows a well-balanced nervous system. A long, straight nose shows a sensitive, nervous nature. A short flat nose reveals an inclination towards rigid thinking.

A red nose indicates the possibility of blood pressure abnormalities – especially high blood pressure. A purple nose may show low blood pressure. If the nose is white, coldness is present in the peripheral areas of the body (i.e. fingers and toes).

Well-developed nostrils show a strong masculine character, courage and determination. On the other hand, less-developed nostrils indicate a feminine nature, sensitivity and gentleness. Overdeveloped nostrils can indicate a tendency towards aggression whereas underdeveloped nostrils show a lack of vitality.

A nose which bends towards the right show that the organs on the right hand side of the body are more active than the organs on the left side. If the nose bends to the left, the organs on the left side are more dominant. Pimples and spots may also appear.

The eyes

Eyebrows

Eyebrows show the history of our development during pregnancy. The early stage of embryonic growth is reflected in the inner section of the eyebrows, middle stage in the middle of the eyebrows and the ends show the last stage of pregnancy. These portions of the eyebrows also show the youth, middle and old age of a person's life.

Space between the eyebrows
The distance between the eyebrows is determined by the food the mother ate during pregnancy.

A narrow distance is caused by over-consumption of animal foods and overcooked vegetables laced with salt. Problems may arise in the liver, pancreas, kidneys and heart. A narrow space can indicate stubbornness, determination and a narrow mind.

A wider space is the result of excessive consumption of milk, sugar, fruits, soft drinks and raw leafy vegetables. The lungs, gall bladder, intestines and bladder may be affected. A wider distance may show indecisiveness, lack of determination and drive, and insecurity.

Angles of the eyebrows
Upward slanting eyebrows reveal a more aggressive nature whereas eyebrows which curve downwards indicate a gentle and understanding character. Peaked eyebrows indicate a person who is physically active but has a gentle nature.

Hair in the eyebrows
The thicker the eyebrows, the more energetic a person is. Long eyebrows indicate a long life whereas short eyebrows show a shorter life – it is interesting to compare the eyebrows with the lifelines on the palm. Broken eyebrows indicate a serious illness has occurred or may occur.

Eyes
The eyes are the mirrors of the soul as well as our health.

Size of the eyes
Small eyes indicate a confidence, determination, strength and vitality. If they are abnormally small, however, there may be an aggressive tendency.

Larger eyes reveal sensitivity and gentleness. Abnormally large eyes indicate a tendency towards nervous disorders, shyness and lack of confidence.

Space between the eyes
A short distance between the eyes as in the case of the eyebrows may reveal stubbornness, determination and a tendency towards

Areas of the eyebrows

a early pregnancy — youth
b middle part of pregnancy — middle age
c later part of pregnancy — old age

wider space
between the eyebrows

narrow space
between the eyebrows

Angle of the eyebrows

upward slanting
eyebrows

downward curving
eyebrows

figure 7 eyebrows

narrow-mindedness and aggression. A wider space indicates a
more gentle character that is indecisive and slower intellectually.

Around the eyes

A clear, natural skin colour around the eyes indicates excellent
physical and mental health.

Dark colour around the eyes indicates weak functioning
particularly of the kidneys and adrenal exhaustion, but there
may also be weakness in the reproductive organs. Redness
appears around the eyes if the heart and circulatory systems are
overworking. The eyelids may become red in women who suffer
from irregular menstruation when the period is due, together
from nervousness. A yellowing may occur if the liver and gall
bladder are under pressure due to over-consumption of dairy
foods. If pimples appear around the eyes the body is trying to
eliminate foods and drinks that have been consumed in excess.

Bags under the eyes that are watery and swollen show disorders of the kidneys – urination is often frequent. Fatty, swollen eye bags indicate mucous and fat accumulating in the kidney tissues. Fatigue, lethargy, forgetfulness and indecisiveness will be present with both types of eye bag.

The ears

The ears represent the whole body and in particular the kidneys. They reflect the diet eaten during pregnancy. If a balanced diet was eaten throughout pregnancy the ears will span from the level of the eyes to mouth level at the earlobe.

Ears that are positioned high on the head may result in a sharper, more aggressive person and pointed ears indicate a tendency towards aggression and narrow-mindedness.

Generally speaking the bigger the ears, the stronger the constitution. Never complain about your big ears ever again! Small ears usually indicate an individual who looks at the immediate problems rather than the broader picture. Thick ears show broadmindedness whereas thin ears indicate a tendency towards prejudice.

Position of ears

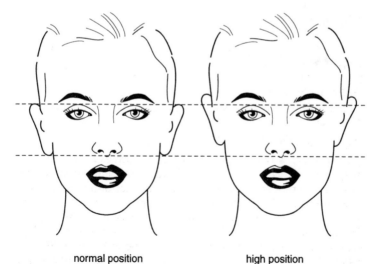

normal position   high position

figure 8 ears

If you look at an ear more closely, three layers become evident. All the organs and glands of the body can be found in the ears. During the Indian head massage treatment, as you massage the ear you are working on approximately 200 points!

The cheeks

The respiratory system is particularly represented on the cheek area as well as the circulatory and digestive systems.

Well-developed, firm cheeks with clear, clean skin and colour indicate excellent respiratory and digestive function. Thinner flesh than normal reflects an under-functioning of the above systems.

Red cheeks, on a physical level, show a tendency towards hypertension (high blood pressure) and, on a mental level, a nervous disposition. White cheeks caused by the over-consumption of dairy foods leads to mucous especially in the lungs. Pimples on the cheeks show mucous is accumulating in the lungs, especially due to high intake of milk.

The mouth

The mouth reflects the condition of the digestive organs – it is, after all, where we put the food and drink that we consume! The upper lip relates to the stomach, the lower lip to the small and large intestines.

Size of the mouth

The size of the mouth has increased over the last few generations and actually indicates degeneration of the physical and mental constitution! This is due to excessive consumption of sugar and sweeteners, coffee and other beverages, fats, tomatoes and potatoes during the pregnancy.

A person with a mouth that is the same width as the nose enjoys excellent physical and mental health. A wide mouth, pre-dominant in modern society, indicates weaker organs and loss of the ability of endurance, resistance and perseverance.

Colour of the lips

Swollen lips reveal digestive disorders. A swollen upper lip indicates stomach problems and an expanded lower lip shows intestinal problems including constipation and diarrhoea. More than seven out of ten people have swollen lower lips. Pinkish-red lips indicate good circulation and sound functioning of the digestive system. However, if the lips are a vivid red this may show high blood pressure or inflammation. White lips reveal poor circulation and perhaps a blood condition such as anaemia.

As you can see it is amazing what the face reveals. Interestingly, some of the features that people now crave for, and indeed even have plastic surgery to create, such as bigger lips, are not necessarily a sign of good health!

By massaging the face and head you are actually working on and improving the functions of every organ of the body. It is most revealing to observe the face prior to your Indian head massage treatment!

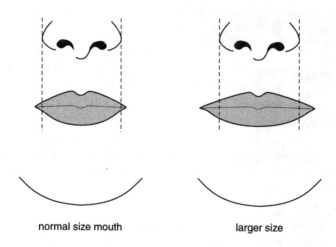

normal size mouth   larger size

figure 9 mouth

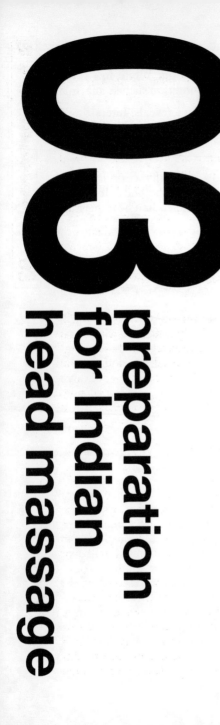

03

preparation for Indian head massage

In this chapter you will learn:

- how to prepare the room for an Indian head massage treatment
- how to prepare yourself
- how to prepare the receiver
- the contraindications to Indian head massage.

Preparation prior to Indian head massage is invaluable. It is important to create a relaxing, tranquil and soothing environment so that both you and your massage partner can enjoy the treatment.

The room

- **Choose a quiet room** where you are unlikely to be disturbed or where interruptions will be minimal. Turn off the telephone or switch on the answerphone. Tell your family and friends that you do not wish to be disturbed for at least half an hour and settle down any pets. Distractions are very disconcerting and if you are worried about being disturbed this will break your concentration and destroy the flow of your massage movements. This is a 'special' time for massage partners – a time to nurture and give them some space and quality time to relax and let go of stress and indulge in a pleasurable experience.
- **Check the temperature of the room.** It should be warm enough so that the recipient can relax but not too warm that it is stuffy. During the treatment, the receiver's body temperature will drop even if he/she has not removed any clothes. You should always think of the comfort of your partner – although you may get rather warm moving around and massaging, your partner will be relaxing. It is impossible to relax if you feel cold and the benefits of the Indian head massage will be lost if the room is not warm enough.

  Ideally the room should not only be pleasantly warm but also well ventilated yet draught-free.
- **Choose soft and subdued lighting for your treatment.** Bright overhead lights beaming down on the receiver's face are not conducive to relaxation and will cause tension around the eyes. If possible, use a dimmer switch if you have one or even better, light some candles. The gentle glow of candlelight can provide the perfect setting. You may find tinted bulbs or sidelights useful and of course natural light is suitable too.
- **Burn some essential oils.** To add an extra special touch to the atmosphere, burn some pure essential oils. These can have a profound effect on the emotions and can encourage deep relaxation, invigorate and increase energy levels or even create a sensual atmosphere. A small, inexpensive clay burner is ideal for diffusing your essential oils and these are readily available and easy to use. Simply put a few teaspoons of water

into the bowl on top of your oil burner and then add a few drops of your favourite essential oil(s). Detailed information on essential oils can be found in *Teach Yourself Aromatherapy*, but here are a few oils that you may wish to try to affect the mood of the receiver.

Deeply relaxing oils
- chamomile
- clary sage
- frankincense
- geranium
- lavender
- sandalwood
- ylang ylang.

Uplifting oils to relieve depression
- bergamot
- geranium
- grapefruit
- lime
- mandarin
- neroli.

Aphrodisiac oils
- jasmine
- neroli
- rose
- ylang ylang.

Oils to improve concentration and clear the mind
- basil
- black pepper
- ginger
- lemon
- peppermint
- rosemary.

Oils to release and clear emotions
- benzoin
- frankincense
- juniper
- linden blossom
- marjoram
- rose.

- **Play some soothing music.** Relaxation music can relax body, mind and spirit and can help to keep conversation to a minimum. Some enjoy listening to natural sounds such as the wind or sea; others prefer dolphin or whale music; some love chants. Check if your partner has any preferences. Some people enjoy silence during the treatment.
- **Place some crystals in the room.** Crystals can greatly enhance the ambience:
  - a piece of purple amethyst will help to absorb any negativity, promote peace and contentment and balance mind, body and spirit
  - rose quartz will encourage love and compassion and create a sense of gentleness and calm
  - clear quartz, which is used extensively for healing by crystal therapists, helps to clear blockages, restore balance and increases energy
  - hematite helps to strengthen our connection with the earth and is useful for grounding the receiver at the end of a treatment.

Place your crystals in a position where you can see them and, if possible, feel their healing vibrations. You can, if you wish, place the crystals around you and your partner as you carry out the treatment.

Equipment

Make sure that you have everything on hand that you may need to perform your Indian head massage. You should not leave the room once you have started your treatment. Here is a checklist:

- **Chair.** A suitable chair is a fairly upright one with quite a low back, preferably without arms. Select a chair which is at comfortable working height – you should be able to reach your partner's head, neck and shoulders without straining or tensing your back. The chair should be low-backed so that the receiver's upper back and shoulders are accessible. The chair should be of a height so that your partner can rest his/her feet firmly on the ground.
- **Cushions/pillows.** Ensure that you have plenty of cushions and pillows on hand to make your partner comfortable. They may wish to place a cushion behind their lower back and you will need a cushion to place on their lap so that they can rest their hands on it. You may also need a pillow for the receiver

to rest their head on while you massage their face.

- **Towels.** If you are using oil in your treatment, you will need a large towel to wrap around your partner. Also have one or two towels to hand to ensure the warmth of the receiver as the treatment progresses.
- **Oils (optional).** You will need a suitable carrier oil and may even wish to make up a suitable essential oil blend prior to the treatment (refer to Chapter 04 for information on oils).
- **Crystals (optional).** You may wish to give the receiver a crystal to hold in each hand while you are treating them. Smooth, polished stones are particularly suitable.
- **Water.** Place some purified water and glasses in the room for use at the end of the session. During the treatment toxins will be released and a glass of purified water will help to flush them out of the system.
- **A large hair clip/hair tie.** While massaging the upper back, shoulders and neck it is helpful to secure long hair on top of the head with a clip.

Personal preparation

- **Clothes.** Wear comfortable, loose-fitting clothes so that you can relax and move easily around your partner. A loose-fitting or short-sleeved T-shirt teamed up with a pair of baggy trousers is ideal, as you will become very warm when giving the treatment. Washable clothes are most practical in case you accidentally spill any oil on your clothes. Make sure that your clothes are freshly laundered.
- **Shoes.** Shoes are optional. You can work barefoot or wear flat or low-heeled shoes or comfortable trainers.

Hygiene

- **Hands.** It is essential that your hands are clean. Always wash them both prior to and after an Indian head massage treatment. Cover any cuts or abrasions that you may have with a plaster.
- **Nails.** Make sure nails are clean, and trim them down as far as possible so that they will not scratch or dig into the receiver. It is advisable not to wear nail polish, as some individuals are allergic to it and could develop a rash. Enamel can also hide dirt!
- **Oral.** Do not eat highly spiced foods such as garlic, or smoke prior to a treatment. You come into close proximity with the

receiver and smells can be off-putting to others. You may need to brush your teeth or use a mouthwash to freshen the breath.

- **Personal.** As you are working in very close proximity to the receiver try to ensure that your body odour is not unpleasant.
- **Hair.** If your hair is long you may find it practical to tie it back.
- **Jewellery.** Remove any jewellery since rings, bracelets and watches can scratch the receiver.

Hand exercises

To perform an Indian head massage effectively it is important that the hands are flexible, strong yet sensitive. The following hand exercises will help to strengthen and mobilize your hands. Perform them whenever you get a free moment, on a daily basis if possible.

1 Hold a small rubber ball in your hand and squeeze and relax your fingers around the ball repeatedly. Now exercise the other hand in the same way.
2 Gently pull and stretch out the thumb and fingers of each hand one by one. Then circle each one carefully.
3 Place your hands face down and shake them out from the wrists as loosely and as rapidly as possible.
4 With fingers relaxed, circle both wrists clockwise and anti-clockwise. You can also perform this movement with your fists clenched.
5 With hands relaxed, bend each joint and slowly close each hand into a fist with the thumb outside the fingers. You can also perform this movement rapidly ensuring that a fist is made each time.
6 Throw out your fingers so that they are separated and extended as far as possible. Repeat at least ten times.
7 Tuck your elbows closely into your waist and rotate your loose wrists and forearms quickly in both directions.
8 Place the palms of your hands together in a prayer position. Rapidly rub your hands together in a backwards and forwards motion. Notice the heat produced by this movement.
9 Practise hacking and cupping on a cushion, remembering to keep your elbows closely tucked in and gradually building up speed.

The following hand exercises will help to increase the sensitivity of your hands:

1 Bring the palms of your hands close to each other so that they are almost touching. Close your eyes and take note of any unusual sensations such as tingling, heat, vibrations or pulsation. Now slowly separate your hands until they are about 5 cm (2 inches) apart. Then return them to the original position and again note any sensations. Now expand the gap to about 10 cm (4 inches) and then to 15 cm (6 inches), all the time observing any reactions.

2 Ask a partner to sit opposite you. Place your hands approximately 5 cm (3 inches) away from his or her body, starting at the head. Move your hands slowly and steadily down the body to scan the energy field. You may feel temperature changes, tingling, vibrations, pulsations or electric shock-type sensations. Repeat this exercise with your hands about 20 cm (8 inches) away from the person to be scanned.

3 Place a coin under a magazine and with your eyes closed try to find the coin by careful palpation of the upper surface of the magazine. If this is too difficult at first, place the coin under a few sheets of paper and then try to sense its position. Gradually increase the thickness of the barrier between your fingers and the coin until you can find the coin under a telephone directory!

4 Place a human hair under a piece of paper and with your eyes closed try to sense it under the page. Once you can do this easily, place the hair under several pages and repeat the exercise.

5 Place a selection of objects made of different materials (e.g. clay, rubber, plastic, metal, wood) in front of you. With your eyes closed pick up each one in turn and feel the different shapes, texture and flexibility of each item.

6 Sit opposite a partner at a table. Ask your partner to rest one or both arms in a relaxed position on the table. Place one of your hands on to your partner's forearm and the other hand on the table. Focus your attention on what you are feeling. Sense the contrast between living tissue and non-living. You may even feel your hand being 'drawn' towards a certain area of the forearm, wrist or upper arm – if there has been an injury at some time this will still manifest in the tissues.

When performing these exercises, ensure that you concentrate fully and use light and slow pressure to get maximum sensory input. Relax your hands as much as possible – rigid, hard hands are not nearly as effective.

By performing these exercises and using massage oils in your Indian head massage, your hands will be softer and suppler than ever before!

State of mind

It is important to spend some time consciously relaxing yourself prior to a treatment. This will enable you to attain a state of peace or tranquillity that is conducive to giving an Indian head massage. Try the following simple relaxation session:

1 Sit comfortably either on the floor or on a chair. It is important to sit upright with your spine straight as this enables your energies to flow freely and helps you to establish a strong connection with the earth.
2 Close your eyes and take a few deep breaths. As you breathe out feel the tension flowing out of your body. On the inhalation feel yourself filling with healing love and light.
3 If you have any tightness in your neck and shoulders or any other part of your body, gently breathe into these areas, melting away any tension.
4 Now that your body is relaxed start to empty your mind of its restless chatter. Focus on a simple word such as 'peace' or 'unity' and keep repeating this word over and over again until your mind becomes quiet and still. If you prefer you can focus on a particular colour until your thoughts fade away.
5 Stay in this state of relaxation for as long as you wish. When you are ready to return, become aware of your body – feel your contact with the earth and wriggle your fingers and toes. Gently open your eyes and notice how relaxed and centred you feel.

This tranquil state of mind and body that you have achieved will be transmitted to the receiver as you work on them. The healing energies will also flow through you, and your intuition and sensitivity will be heightened.

Preparation of the receiver

- **Clothes.** If the receiver wants a massage without oil then he or she should wear a T-shirt. If you are using oil for your treatment (and this is far more therapeutic), your partner should take off his or her upper clothing. It is a good idea to take off the bra or to adjust the bra straps so that the shoulders are bare. Wrap a large towel or a piece of natural fabric around the chest.

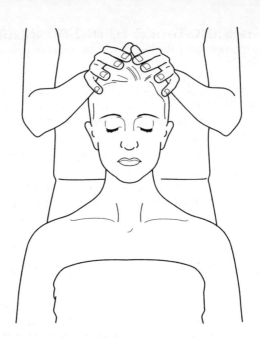

figure 10 connecting

- **Jewellery.** Ask your partner to remove any jewellery such as necklaces, earrings and nose rings or other facial piercings.
- **Glasses.** Take off spectacles.
- **Hair.** Brush through the hair so that during the treatment you will not pull on any tangles. If the hair is long, use a clip to tie it up while you are working on the upper back, shoulders and neck.
- **Make-up.** Remove face make-up so that optimum benefits can be obtained from the oil during the facial massage.
- **Position.** Seat the receiver comfortably in a chair. Ask the receiver to remove shoes and make sure that their legs are uncrossed and that their feet are placed on the ground. Place a pillow on their lap and ask them to rest their hands lightly on it. You may offer your partner a crystal to hold, one in each hand.
- **Check for contraindications.** Check that there are no reasons why you should not carry out an Indian head massage treatment (see below for details).
- **Explain** to the receiver briefly what Indian head massage is, what the treatment involves and what the benefits are.

Contraindications to Indian head massage

Contraindications are disorders or any other factors which indicate that you should not perform an Indian head massage treatment. You should check for these contraindications prior to giving a massage because you do not wish to aggravate any condition.

Massage is one of the most natural, non-invasive and safe therapies. There are only a limited number of cases when advice should be sought prior to the treatment or extra care needs to be taken. If you have any doubts, seek the advice of a medically qualified doctor or a professional, experienced head massage therapist.

When not to perform Indian head massage

Fever

If the receiver has a high temperature or fever, you should wait until it has subsided. A raised temperature indicates that the body is already fighting off infection and that its defence mechanisms have been activated. An Indian head massage may introduce toxins into a system that already has enough to contend with!

Thrombosis/embolism

Thrombosis or embolism (blood clot) is a contraindication to treatment. There is a risk that the blood clot could become detached and be carried to another part of the body where it could obstruct the flow of blood to a vital organ. If the embolus is large enough to cause a complete blockage, this could result in immediate death. If there is a history of thrombosis, ask for the advice of the doctor before giving a treatment.

Recent haemorrhage

A haemorrhage is excessive bleeding which may be either internal or external. Massage is obviously inadvisable.

Infectious/contagious diseases

If the receiver has an infectious disease such as chicken pox, measles, flu, impetigo or scabies, massage should be avoided. You do not want to aggravate the condition or spread it to yourself or to other people. Some of the most common skin diseases that may be encountered on the head or neck include:

- **Impetigo.** A highly infectious and contagious disease caused by streptococcal and staphylococcal bacteria. It is most commonly found on the face near the mouth, nose and around the ears, but it may appear on the scalp. It is indicated by blisters, usually in groups, which burst and then dry leading to the formation of yellow crusts.
- **Herpes simplex (cold sores).** This virus is present in approximately 90 per cent of the population and may be activated by stress, ill health or sunlight. It is commonly found around the lips and begins as an itching sensation followed by the appearance of small blisters around the mouth. These weep and form crusts and persist for approximately two to three weeks.
- **Tinea capitis (ringworm of the scalp).** Tinea capitis is a fungal infection that appears as circular patches that may look red and scaly and can itch (tinea corporis is ringworm of the body).
- **Pediculosis capitis (head lice).** The head louse is a small parasite that feeds on blood from the scalp. Nits are found in the hair close to the scalp and the person will complain of itching. The scalp may look red due to itching.

N.B. Non-infectious, non-contagious skin conditions include psoriasis, eczema, dermatitis, dandruff and alopecia (hair loss). If the affected areas are sensitive or weeping, however, treat them as a local contraindication.

Local areas of infection

If the receiver has a local area of infection such as a boil, carbuncle, conjunctivitis or a stye, that area only should be avoided. Boils and carbuncles are commonly found on the back of the neck, contain pus and can be very painful and are infectious. Conjunctivitis is an inflammation of the lining of the eyelid where the eye becomes red, swollen and discharges. It is easily spread from one eye to the other. Styes result from infected hair follicles.

Recent head/neck injury

If the receiver has recently sustained an injury such as a whiplash or a recent blow to the head, Indian head massage is inadvisable. Massage could exacerbate the condition and may even make it worse by increasing the inflammation and pain.

Recent head/neck surgery

If the receiver has recently undergone surgery to the head or neck, avoid massage since it may interfere with the healing process. Massage on recent scars could cause tissue damage, pain, and delay healing. Always wait until the doctor has pronounced complete recovery. However, if the surgery is not recent, massage is excellent for reducing scar tissue, decreasing pain and increasing mobility.

Intoxication

If the receiver is under the influence of alcohol, the increase of blood flow to the head could result in nausea and dizziness. Anyone under the influence of drugs should also not be treated.

Swelling/inflammation

Any swollen or inflamed area should be avoided due to the risk of aggravation.

Migraine attack

Although Indian head massage is an excellent way of preventing a migraine attack, particularly if it is stress-related, never try to carry out a treatment during an attack. The receiver may be nauseous, dizzy, experience visual disturbances and severe pain, and may even vomit.

Heart conditions/circulatory disorders

If your massage partner is suffering from a severe heart condition or very high or very low blood pressure then seek advice from their doctor and exercise caution. Massage is highly effective for lowering the blood pressure, but patients on anti-hypersensitive medications may be prone to feeling dizzy and light-headed after the treatment. They should always get up slowly.

Cuts, bruises, abrasions etc.

If a local area of skin is damaged or open, then avoid the area. Cuts, wounds, abrasions, bruises, moles, blisters, areas of sensitivity, sunburn, veins, bites, stings and blisters are all local contraindications.

Lumps/bumps

If the receiver has any undiagnosed lumps or bumps they should be referred to their doctor for diagnosis. Suspicious moles should also be investigated.

Disorders of the nervous system

If the receiver suffers from a dysfunction of the nervous system such as Parkinson's disease, cerebral palsy, multiple sclerosis or epilepsy, check with the doctor and exercise caution. A gentle treatment is very beneficial and can relieve spasm and rigidity. In the case of epilepsy, the incidence of attacks may be reduced.

Diabetes

Pressure should be very light as diabetics may suffer with a loss of sensory function and will be unable to give you accurate feedback.

Osteoporosis

Only light and gentle movements are indicated since the bones are brittle and more prone to fracture.

Myalgic encephalomyelitis (ME)

Use only relaxing movements on those who suffer from chronic fatigue. If patients are treated with care, energy levels can show a remarkable improvement the day after treatment.

Cancer

Massage is very beneficial for cancer sufferers. Radiotherapy sites and tumour sites, however, should be avoided.

Frailty

A light pressure only should be used.

Pregnancy

Many problems in pregnancy can be alleviated by Indian head massage. Special care should be taken to ensure the comfort of the mother-to-be. In the first trimester, keep movements light and gentle. Be aware of any complications such as high blood pressure and gestational diabetes, which could develop during pregnancy.

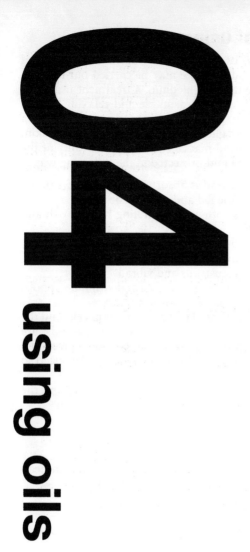

04
using oils

In this chapter you will learn:

- the benefits of using oils
- the properties and indications of carrier oils
- the top ten essential oils for the hair and skin
- how to select the appropriate oils and prepare a blend.

The benefits of using oils

In India, oils are always used in head massage on both men and women. Although a head massage may be carried out through the clothes without the use of a medium, a treatment using oils is far more therapeutic, more pleasurable and relaxing for the receiver. It is also easier to give an Indian head massage, using a medium as your hands can glide smoothly over the hair and skin. If oil is used for Indian head massage, the natural beauty of the skin and hair is promoted and protected in the following ways:

- oil massaged on to the head is absorbed into the roots of the hair so that it is strengthened and nourished
- the skin of the scalp is softened, promoting hair growth and slowing down hair loss
- the sebaceous glands are activated, encouraging the production of sebum, which is the hairs' natural moisturizer, the hair becomes shiny, lustrous and vibrant
- hair is protected from the harsh sun, sea and swimming pools, which cause the hair to become brittle and dry
- the use of oil encourages the shedding of old skin cells and the regeneration of new skin cells – some essential oils are particularly effective; a fresh, glowing complexion is promoted
- the sebaceous glands improve in function and are balanced so that the skin becomes soft and supple
- oil can help to cleanse the pores thoroughly, flushing out the toxins and encouraging a healthy, flawless complexion.

Choosing a carrier oil

There are a wide range of oils that are suitable for Indian head massage. They are known as carrier, base or fixed oils.

The carrier oil chosen should be cold-pressed since oils produced by the process of 'hot extraction' may be cheaper but are of an inferior quality. The oil you choose should be unrefined and untreated by chemicals because the more highly processed an oil is the less vitamin content will be retained. Try to find carrier oils which are free of additives (colour is often added) as these can cause allergies. In short, choose cold-pressed, unrefined, additive-free base oils for best results. Mineral oil such as commercial baby oil is unsuitable. It tends to clog the pores and lacks the nutritional constituents of the vegetable oils which nourish the skin. The reason that mineral oil is so favoured by the cosmetics industry is because it does not become rancid. The most popular carrier oils in Indian head massage are **coconut, mustard, olive, sesame** and **sweet almond oil.**

Coconut oil – *cocos nucifera*

Coconut oil is widely used in southern India, especially in the spring. It is thought to keep the head cool and is particularly recommended for women. Coconut oil is used a great deal for cosmetics, soaps and hair preparations. It has to be subjected to heat in order to provide a workable oil. It is a light–medium oil, suitable for all skin and hair types. Coconut oil is very moisturizing for the hair and skin. Solid at room temperature, coconut oil liquefies when warmed. Place your bottle of coconut oil in a jug of hot water or stand it near a radiator prior to use.

Uses
- all skin and hair types
- dry, chapped or sunburnt skin
- dry, brittle hair
- chemically treated hair
- protection from the sun.

Special precautions
- Take care with hypersensitive skin

Mustard oil – *brassica nigra*

Mustard oil is widely used in India, particularly in the Northwest. It is especially recommended in the winter months due to the hot, warming sensation it creates, and it is used extensively for men. In Ayurvedic medicine, the crushed seeds are used as an aid to digestion and to alleviate stomach disorders.

Mustard oil has a very powerful pungent aroma and it is a thick, heavy massage oil. Mustard oil is renowned for its ability to increase body heat. Highly suitable for poor circulation, muscular aches, joint stiffness, pains and swellings and congestion, it is a stimulating carrier oil.

Uses:
- generating heat
- stimulating
- muscular tension
- relieving pain
- joint stiffness.

Special precautions
- take care with sensitive skins and scalps
- do not use essential oil of mustard.

Olive oil – *olea europaea*

Olive oil is widely available in the West and is used extensively for cooking and healing. Its ability to protect against heart disease is well known. Olive oil should only be used if it is virgin and cold-pressed. It has rather a pungent smell. Olive oil has excellent moisturizing properties and is soothing and penetrative.

Uses
- dry, damaged brittle hair
- dry skin
- inflamed skin and scalp
- swellings
- detox regimes
- rheumatism
- muscular pain and stiffness.

Special precautions
- none – olive oil is very safe.

Sesame oil – *sesamum indicum*

This is possibly the most popular carrier oil in India used for Indian head massage. Sesame oil is used extensively in Ayurvedic medicine. It is rich in minerals such as iron, calcium and phosphorus as well as vitamins A and E, protein and lecithin. Vitamin A acts to protect the skin and vitamin E soothes and heals.

Sesame oil is fairly viscous and has quite a strong odour which does not appeal to everyone. Its main claim to fame is its ability to prevent the hair from turning grey and to restore the hair to its natural colour. Sesame oil is particularly popular in India as a summer oil. It does provide some protection from the rays of the sun.

Uses
- all skin and hair types, especially dry
- eczema, psoriasis
- sun protection
- swelling
- muscular pains
- prevents greyness and restores hair colour.

Special precautions
- Take care with highly sensitive skin.

Sweet almond oil – *prunus amygdalus*

Sweet almond oil is one of the most widely used in the West and is very much favoured by the beauty industry. It is reputed to have been used by Napoleon's wife, Josephine. Extracted by cold pressing from the kernels of the sweet almond, it is rich in vitamins, protein and unsaturated fatty acids. Sweet almond is a yellow oil, low in odour and it is not too thick, sticky or heavy. This makes it a particularly suitable oil for massage.

Easily absorbed, sweet almond oil is excellent for moisturizing dry skin and for dry hair that has been chemically treated. It is often used in moisturizers and hair conditioners.

Uses
- all skin types, particularly dry, sensitive, inflamed or prematurely aged skin
- itching of the skin or scalp
- eczema
- easing muscular pain and stiffness.

Special precautions
- do not use bitter almond oil.

Other suitable carrier oils

The oils already described are the most popular for Indian head massage. However, there are many other suitable carrier oils and it is a matter of personal preference. Below is a brief description of other recommended base oils.

Apricot kernel – *prunus armenica*

Suitable for all skin types, especially prematurely aged, dry, inflamed or sensitive. A moisturizing oil for the hair.

Avocado oil – *persea americana*

A penetrative carrier oil which is excellent for dry, dehydrated, sun-damaged skin and eczema. Avocado oil is a thick, dark green oil which is useful for dry, brittle, chemically treated hair.

Borage seed oil – *borago officinalis*

A pale yellow oil rich in GLA (gamma linoleic acid), vitamins and minerals. Its rejuvenating properties and ability to fight dehydration make it suitable for dry, damaged, mature skin that has lost elasticity. Borage will help dry, permed hair.

Calendula oil – *calendula officinalis*

Renowned for its anti-inflammatory, healing and soothing properties, calendula oil is highly beneficial for all skin disorders and scalp problems especially where there is hypersensitivity.

Carrot oil – *daucus carota*

Rejuvenating and regenerative, carrot oil is thought to delay the process of ageing. Carrot oil is also useful for dry, itchy skins and scalps.

Corn oil – *zea mays*

May be used on all types of skin and hair, although it is used mainly for cooking.

Evening primrose oil – *oenothera biennis*

Useful for all types of skin and hair. Particularly good for the treatment of dry, sensitive and allergic type skin problems such as eczema. A wonderful oil for nourishing the hair and for premature ageing.

Grapeseed oil – *vitis vinifera*

Almost colourless and odourless, which accounts for its popularity. It can be used for all types of hair and skin.

Hazlenut oil – *corylus avellana*

An amber–yellow oil that penetrates deeply and has a slight astringent action. Recommended for moisturizing and protecting the hair and skin from sun damage.

Hypericum oil (St John's Wort) – *hypericum perforatum*

A ruby red oil that is excellent for inflamed skins and scalps. It also eases aches and pains.

Jojoba oil – *simmondsia chinensis*

A particular favourite for the skin and hair – more expensive but worth it! Jojoba is ideal for the face as it nourishes, moisturizes and penetrates deeply. Jojoba imparts a silky feel to the skin. It helps damaged, dry brittle hair, protecting and renewing, and adding a glossy shine.

Macadamia nut oil – *macadamia integrifolia*

Helpful for dry, sun damaged and prematurely aged skins. Suitable for dry, brittle hair.

Peach kernel oil – *prunus persica*

Beneficial for everyone but particularly effective as an emollient for dry, mature skin, helping to increase elasticity. Suitable for treating dry and damaged hair.

Peanut oil – *arachis hypogeae*

Peanut oil can be used on all types of skin and hair but it does have a very distinctive, heavy odour.

Rosehip oil – *rosa rugosa*

This oil is a most effective treatment for skin problems. It is a tissue regenerator making it extremely beneficial for prematurely aged skin.

Safflower oil – *carthamus tinctorius*

Safflower oil can be applied to all types of hair and skin, especially where there is redness and inflammation. Unfortunately, it is not a very stable oil and therefore becomes rancid.

Soya bean oil – *glycine soja*

This pale yellow oil is useful for all types of hair and skin.

Sunflower oil – *helianthus annus*

It is suitable for all skin types and has a light texture. Pleasant to use the skin is left with a smooth, soft, non-greasy feel.

Wheatgerm oil – *triticum vulgare*

A rich orangey–brown colour, wheatgerm is high in vitamin E. It will improve dry, flaky, itchy, peeling skin since it is so nourishing. Wheatgerm will strengthen dry and brittle hair.

Other carrier oils traditionally used in India

The following oils are widely used in India in the treatment of the hair and the skin. Although you will not find these oils in chemists and department stores, they can be found in Indian supermarkets. Do make sure that you only buy the Indian oils in small quantities. Some can have an unpleasant aroma and may be too sticky or watery. If you want the authentic touch experiment with some of these.

Amla oil – *emblica officinalis*

Amla is the edible fruit of a small leafy tree that grows throughout India. The amla fruit is one of the richest sources of vitamin C. In fact, it contains approximately 20 times the vitamin C content of an orange. Medicinally the fruit has been used to treat burning sensations anywhere in the body as well as many digestive disorders such as dyspepsia, constipation, diarrhoea, dysentery and ulcers. In colonial times, the British named it the 'Indian Gooseberry'. It is used to make jams and chutneys in India. To prepare the oil, dried amla berries are soaked in coconut oil for several days. The filtered and purified oil is known as 'amla' oil. Amla oil is used extensively for treating the hair and is one of the world's oldest, natural hair conditioners. It is customary to apply a small amount of amla oil to the hair after washing. This promotes the growth of healthy hair and gives the hair a natural shine. Amla rejuvenates dull and damaged hair and is thought to prevent premature greying. The oil is not only a tonic for the hair but also a general tonic for improving physical and mental well-being.

Bhringaraj oil – *eclipta alba*

The bhringaraj is found all over India and in Ayurvedic medicine is undoubtedly one of the main herbs for the hair. It also has a reputation for anti-ageing and is popularly used to enhance the memory.

Bhringaraj hair oil is commonly prepared by boiling the fresh leaves with either sesame or coconut oil. The resulting blend is believed to promote black and luxuriant hair since it removes greying, balding and makes the hair darker. Bhringaraj is also used for skin conditions.

Brahmi oil – *bacopa monnieri*

Brahmi is used medicinally in India as a tonic for the nervous system for those suffering from anxiety and emotional exhaustion.

As a hair oil, brahmi promotes hair growth as well as improving the memory and dispelling mental fatigue.

Neem oil – *azadirachta indica*

Early Sanskrit medical writings refer to the benefits of neem and, since ancient times, it has been associated with healing in India. Modern research seems to indicate that in the future neem will be used much more widely in the treatment of many diseases. Every part of the neem tree is used for healing – the bark, root, leaves, flowers and seeds.

Neem oil is prepared by crushing the seeds. The resulting oil is antibacterial, antiviral, antifungal and antiparasitic, and is added to toiletries, toothpaste, and skin and hair products.

It is particularly good for relieving itching and irritation, whether of the scalp or of the skin. Neem is also excellent for the treatment of head lice. It should be used in up to a 10 per cent dilution.

Shikakai oil – *acacia concinna*

This shrub-like tree grows in central India and for centuries Indians have used its pod-like fruit to clean their hair. They collected, dried and ground this pod into powder and used it on the hair to promote hair growth and prevent dandruff. 'Shikakai' literally translates as 'fruit for the hair'.

The dried powdered fruit is sold in packages throughout India and it is mixed with water to make a paste which acts as a gentle shampoo and de-tangler.

Shikakai oil has many beneficial properties when used in Indian head massage. It promotes lustrous, long hair and helps to prevent dandruff and soothes a dry, itchy scalp.

Other Indian herbs used for the hair include:

- baheda – hair tonic
- bakuchi – hair growth
- ghritkumari – promotes hair growth and prevents hair loss
- kalonji – hair growth
- kuth – prevents baldness
- mendhi – hair tonic and conditioner
- reetha (soap nut) – a hair tonic.

Pure essential oils

Although carrier oils can be used on their own for the purposes of Indian head massage, the addition of essential oils can enhance your treatment enormously. Pure essential oils have a profound effect on the emotions and they can successfully treat a wide range of skin and hair problems too.

Preparing an oil blend

Essential oils are highly concentrated in their pure state and must be blended with a carrier oil. This vegetable, nut or seed oil must be cold-pressed, unrefined and additive-free. Mineral oil, such as commercial baby oil, is not really suitable since it tends to clog the pores and prevents the skin from breathing. Sweet almond, apricot kernel and peach kernel are particularly recommended since they are suitable for all skin types, are not too heavy or thick to work with and do not have a strong odour.

A teaspoon holds about 5 ml of carrier oil. If you blend 10 ml (two teaspoons), there should be plenty left over for the receiver to use between treatments. For your treatment blend just add three drops of essential oil to 10 ml (two teaspoons) of carrier oil.

If you wish to make up a larger quantity for daily use between treatments, you will need to store your blend in an amber glass bottle since essential oils are damaged by ultra-violet light. A blend will keep for about three to six months if it is stored like this away from sunlight. The appropriate dilutions are as follows:

- three drops of essential oil to 10 ml (two teaspoons) of carrier oil
- six drops of essential oil to 20 ml of carrier oil
- fifteen drops of essential oil to 50 ml of carrier oil
- thirty drops of essential oil to 100 ml of carrier oil

Top ten essential oils for the hair and skin

There are hundreds of essential oils and a professional aroma-therapist will usually use about 50–60. However, to keep it simple, avoid confusion and to save you money, we have chosen ten essential oils which are most useful for the hair and skin. For detailed information on essential oils please refer to *Teach Yourself Aromatherapy*. A brief description of the aroma is also included (if you don't like the smell it won't do any good!) as well as an indication of the effects of the essential oil on your mood. Have fun!

1 bergamot
2 carrot seed
3 chamomile
4 frankincense
5 geranium
6 lavender
7 lemon
8 rose
9 rosemary
10 tea tree.

Bergamot – *citrus bergamia*

- **Aroma.** Light, fresh, citrus.
- **Effects on mood.** Sedative yet uplifting.
- **Hair – use for:** Head lice; oily hair.
- **Skin – use for:** Acne; eczema; oily and open pores; psoriasis.
- **Special precautions.** Do not apply prior to sunbathing because it accelerates sun tanning.

Carrot seed – *daucus carota*

- **Aroma.** Sharp, pungent.
- **Effects on mood.** Revitalizing, stimulating, tonic.
- **Hair – use for:** Dandruff; dry hair.
- **Skin – use for:** Acne; dry skin; mature skin; rejuvenation; scars; wrinkles.
- **Special precautions.** None.

Chamomile (Roman) – *anthemis nobilis*

- **Aroma.** Warm, sweet, floral, aromatic.
- **Effects on mood.** Balancing, calming, soothing.
- **Hair – use for:** Dandruff; hair loss; sensitive scalp.
- **Skin – use for:** Acne; allergic skin; broken capillaries; dry skin; eczema; inflamed, irritated skin; sensitive skin.
- **Special precautions.** None.

Frankincense – *boswellia carterii*

- **Aroma.** Woody, spicy, balsamic, heady.
- **Effects on mood.** Elevating, healing, rejuvenating.
- **Hair – use for:** Dry hair; loss of hair; oily hair.
- **Skin – use for:** Ageing skin; broken capillaries; combination skin; dry skin; mature skin; oily skin; rejuvenation; scars; wrinkles.
- **Special precautions.** None.

Geranium – *pelargonium graveolens*

- **Aroma.** Sweet, rosy.
- **Effects on mood.** Antidepressant, healing, uplifting.
- **Hair – use for:** Dry hair; head lice; loss of hair; oily hair.
- **Skin – use for:** Acne; combination skin; dry skin; eczema; inflamed, irritated skin; mature skin; oily skin; sensitive skin.
- **Special precautions.** None.

Lavender – *lavendula augustifolia/vera/officinalis*

- **Aroma.** Sweet, floral.
- **Effects on mood.** Antidepressant, balancing, calming.
- **Hair – use for:** Dandruff; dry hair; head lice; loss of hair; sensitive scalp.
- **Skin – use for:** Acne; ageing skin; allergic skin; combination skin; dry skin; eczema; inflamed, irritated skin; mature skin; oily skin; psoriasis; rejuvenation; sensitive skin.
- **Special precautions:** None.

Lemon – *citrus limonum*

- **Aroma.** Clean, fruity, refreshing, sharp.
- **Effects on mood.** Uplifting, tonic.
- **Hair – use for:** Dandruff; head lice; oily hair.
- **Skin – use for:** Acne; ageing skin; broken capillaries; mature skin; oily skin; wrinkles.
- **Special precautions.** Avoid strong sunlight immediately after treatment.

Rose – *rosa damascena/rosa centifolia*

- **Aroma.** Sweet, heady, heavenly, intoxicating.
- **Effects on mood.** Balancing, encourages positivity, uplifting.
- **Hair – use for:** Dry hair; inflamed, irritated scalp; sensitive scalp.
- **Skin – use for:** Ageing skin; broken capillaries; dry skin; inflamed, red, irritated skin; mature skin; rejuvenating; sensitive skin; wrinkles.
- **Special precautions.** None.

Rosemary – *rosmarinus officinalis*

- **Aroma.** Clean, strong, slightly camphoraceous.
- **Effects on mood.** Enlivening, restorative, stimulating.
- **Hair – use for:** Dry hair; head lice; loss of hair; oily hair.
- **Skin – use for:** Acne; ageing skin; wrinkles.
- **Special precautions.** Do not use extensively in the first stages of pregnancy or on those with epilepsy.

Tea tree – melaleuca alternifolia

- **Aroma.** Sharp, strong, medicinal.
- **Effects on mood.** Stimulating.
- **Hair – use for:** Dandruff; head lice; infections of the scalp; oily hair.
- **Skin – use for:** acne; oily skin; psoriasis.
- **Special precautions.** None.

For best results from your Indian head massage, try to select the most appropriate blend. You may decide to use one essential oil or two or three essential oils for your blend. It does not matter as long as you follow the guidelines on pages 50–51.

Example 1

Your massage partner has dry hair and a sensitive scalp. Her skin is also dry, mature and in need of rejuvenation. Suitable oils to choose for her **hair** would be: carrot seed, chamomile, frankincense, geranium, lavender, rose. Suitable oils to choose for her **skin** would be: carrot seed, frankincense, geranium, lavender, rose.

There are many possible blends to choose from. You may decide to select just one essential oil from the lists above, for example, carrot seed. Therefore, you would mix three drops of carrot seed to 10 ml of carrier oil.

If you decide to select three essential oils, a possible blend could be:

One drop frankincense
One drop geranium   Diluted in
One drop rose   10 ml
                           carrier oil

Example 2

Your massage partner has an oily scalp and is beginning to lose his hair. He has a tendency towards acne. Suitable oils to choose for his **hair** would be: frankincense, geranium, rosemary. Suitable oils to choose for his **skin** would be: bergamot, carrot seed, chamomile, geranium, lavender, lemon, rosemary, tea tree.

A possible combination of essential oils could be:

One drop geranium
One drop lemon   Diluted in
One drop rosemary   10 ml
                           carrier oil

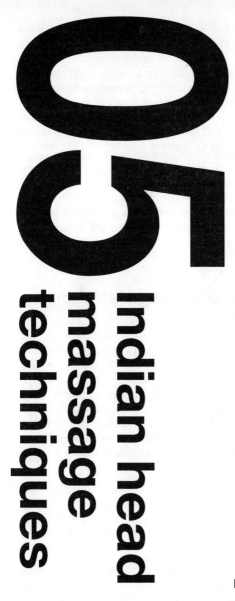

05

Indian head massage techniques

In this chapter you will learn:

- how to perform the basic techniques of Indian head massage
- the benefits of each technique.

The therapeutic massage techniques employed for Indian head massage are very simple yet highly effective. By following the step-by-step instructions, you will soon familiarize yourself with the basic movements. If you feel clumsy at first, don't worry – everyone has a natural instinctive ability to massage. You will be surprised at how quickly your massage strokes will start to flow. As your confidence grows you will find that you naturally begin to develop your own particular style. Practise as often as you can – there will be no shortage of volunteers.

All the techniques in the chapter will be performed with your partner in the seated position as described on page 31. The massage may be practised through the clothes or with the use of a massage medium. An Indian head massage treatment is a far more therapeutic and pleasurable experience if oil is used, and the lubricant enables you to glide smoothly over the skin so that your movements flow freely.

Technique one – effleurage/stroking

Effleurage is one of the principal techniques used in Indian head massage. It is a stroking movement that signals both the beginning and the end of a massage. Effleurage is also a connecting or a link movement that facilitates the flow from one technique to the next. It is the receiver's introduction to massage and allows them to get used to the sensation of touch. It enables the giver to apply the massage medium evenly to the receiver's body and to accustom the hands to the contours of the body. These initial movements establish a sense of trust between giver and receiver as your massage partner melts into a deep state of relaxation.

Effleurage may be performed slowly or briskly. Gentle, slow effleurage has a soothing and relaxing effect. It has a calming, sedative, soporific effect on both body and mind. Brisk effleurage is energizing, enlivening and revitalizing, and banishes tiredness and lethargy.

In Indian head massage a combination of slow, gentle stroking and brisk, energetic effleurage is used in a treatment. To perform effleurage usually the palm of one or both hands is used. However, on smaller areas like the face, the pads of the fingers may be used and on larger areas such as across the top of the shoulders, the forearms may be employed.

Pressure can be superficial or deep depending on the effect that you wish to achieve. As you practise the techniques, always ask your massage partner for feedback. Let the receiver guide you as to how much pressure you should use. Some people find a light pressure ticklish or irritating, others find deep pressure uncomfortable. Asking for feedback will enable you to judge how much pressure you should use.

Let us practise effleurage on the upper back. Seat your partner comfortably on a chair with their legs uncrossed and feet flat on the floor. Stand squarely behind the receiver. If they have long hair ask them to clip it up.

1 Pour a small amount of oil into the palm of one of your hands and rub your hands together so that your palms and fingers and the oil is warmed.
2 Place both hands, palms down, one on each side of the receiver's back, level with the bottom of the shoulder blades. Your fingers should be facing upwards.
3 Use the palmar surface of both hands simultaneously to stroke up the back and across the upper back and shoulders. Mould your hands to the contours of the body. Apply firm rhythmic pressure on the upward stroke yet glide back to your starting point with a feather-light touch. Start with a light pressure and then gradually start to make it firmer. Experiment with different depths of pressure. Repeat the effleurage until the muscles feel relaxed and begin to soften.

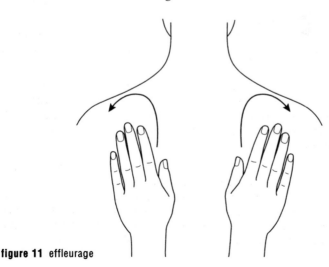

figure 11 effleurage

Benefits of effleurage/stroking

- begins and ends an Indian head massage
- spreads the oil evenly
- acts as a link between techniques
- establishes a relationship of trust
- accustoms your hands to the receiver's body
- familiarizes the receiver with your touch
- enables you to gauge the amount of pressure to apply
- induces well-being
- improves circulation
- increases lymph flow thus aiding the elimination of toxins
- soothes the sensory nerve endings, inducing a deep sense of relaxation throughout the whole body, relieving stress and strain
- prepares the body for deeper movements
- encourages the removal of dead skin cells, encouraging new cell growth and a glowing complexion
- stimulates the sweat glands to produce more sweat so that the skin is purified
- stimulates the sebaceous glands to secrete more sebum so that the skin becomes smooth and supple
- hair becomes glossy, shiny and healthy due to stimulation of the sebaceous glands
- relaxes tense muscles helping to relieve aches and pains, headaches etc.
- brisk effleurage enlivens and revitalizes the receiver.

Points to observe

- do not lose contact
- use your whole hand – not just the fingertips
- relax your hands
- avoid jerky movements – effleurage should be rhythmic, smooth and even
- do not use any pressure on the downward stroke. Return with a feather-light touch
- use more oil on a hairy person.

Technique two – friction

Frictions are deep, penetrating movements that are excellent for finding and breaking down the knots and nodules that accumulate due to stress and tension. This technique is particularly useful for working around the shoulder blades and on either side of the spine.

Friction is usually performed with the balls of the thumbs. However, the pads of the fingers, the knuckles, heels of the hands or even the elbows may be employed. As the small, deep, circular movements are performed the muscle can be moved against the bone. The pressure is gradually increased as you penetrate deeper and deeper into the tissues.

We will practise friction on the upper back.

1 Position yourself squarely behind the receiver as before.
2 Place the pads of the thumbs, one on either side of the receiver's spine, level with the bottom of the shoulder blades.
3 Perform small, deep, penetrating outward circular movements working up the back towards the neck area. Glide gently back to your starting position with a feather-light touch. Repeat the frictions several times to try to pinpoint a tight, knotty area.
4 When you have pinpointed an area of tension, apply extra friction movements gradually increasing the pressure. Use your body weight to penetrate into the deeper tissues. Try placing one thumb on top of the other to achieve a deeper effect. Your partner will feel a great sense of relief as the muscular tension dissipates. It is important when performing friction to be guided by your partner as to how much pressure

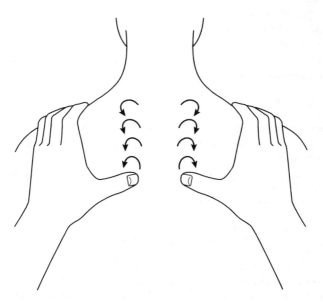

figure 12 friction on the back

to use. If your partner experiences discomfort then decrease your pressure slightly. Pressure should be firm yet not painful.

5 When you have finished your friction movements, soothe down the area with effleurage. This will relax the receiver and also help to disperse any toxins that have been released.

Benefits of friction

- breaks down knots and nodules
- increases circulation to local areas bringing with it oxygen and nutrients
- improves lymph flow thus speeding up the elimination of waste products
- provides analgesia (pain relief)
- breaks down fatty deposits
- helps break down old scar tissue.

Points to observe

- use the pads of the thumbs only, not the tips, to avoid digging the nails in
- ensure you are moving the tissues under the skin and not just the skin
- work more deeply into the tissues gradually
- do not over-treat any problem areas as this could lead to soreness
- take care not to use too much oil otherwise your thumbs will slip and slide and you will find it very difficult to pinpoint troublesome areas
- do not hunch your shoulders with the effort
- always finish with effleurage.

Friction vs rubbing

Friction is different from the movement known as 'rubbing'. Rubbing is a much lighter technique whereby your hands move over the surface of the skin. You rub over the surface of the skin rather than moving muscle over bone as with friction.

Technique three – petrissage

The word petrissage is derived from the French *pétrir* which means 'to knead'. There are many different types of petrissage including **picking up**, **squeezing**, **rolling** and **wringing**. As the name implies the action is rather like kneading dough – if you are good at making bread then you will quickly become an expert!

Petrissage is a more vigorous movement than effleurage and enables you to work deeply into the muscles. The soft tissues are firmly picked up and lifted from the underlying structures, compressed and then released. The whole hand is used to perform petrissage rather than just the fingers and the thumbs. Sometimes the heels of the hand may be used.

Petrissage may be performed on every part of the body except for the face. It is particularly suitable and effective for the fleshy areas of the body such as across the top of the shoulders. This is the area where you will practise the technique.

1 Position yourself squarely behind the receiver as before.
2 Place your hands, palms downward, one on top of the each of the receiver's shoulders. Your thumbs should be at the back of the shoulders and your fingers over the tops of the shoulders.
3 **Pick up, squeeze and release.** Grasp the muscles (not the skin) firmly with both hands and pick up, squeeze and release the muscles. Make sure you are not pinching the flesh between your fingers and thumbs – it is the palms of the hands that do most of the work.
  For extra practice you may continue this technique down the upper arms. Picking up and squeezing is very effective for releasing muscle spasm. Repeat this technique until you feel the soft tissues warm up and soften.

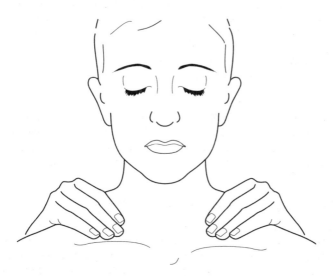

figure 13 pick up, squeeze and release the shoulder muscles

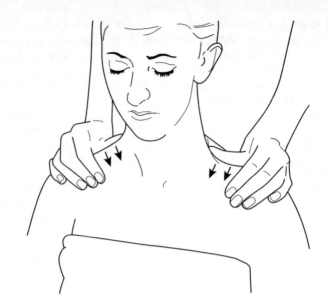

figure 14 thumb pushes on the shoulders

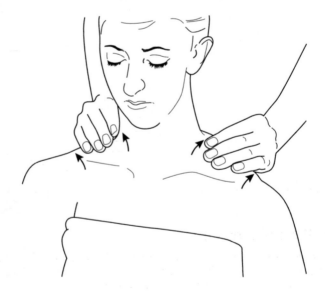

figure 15 finger pulls on the shoulders

4 **Pick up and roll**
   a *Thumb pushes.* With your hands in the same position, push your thumbs forwards towards the fingers. Gently roll the tissues towards the fingers, working all across the top of the shoulders. You may also try performing this action with the heels of your hands instead of your thumbs. This is particularly effective if you are working over broad shoulders.
   b *Finger pulls.* Still in the same position this time use your fingers to pull back the muscles towards your thumbs. Repeat this action across the entire length of the shoulders.
5 **Wringing.** This is a variation on picking up. It is picking up with a twist! Stand behind the shoulder you wish to work on. Place both hands, palms downward, on top of one of the receiver's shoulders. Use one hand to pick up the muscle, squeeze it and pull it towards you. Then repeat the procedure using the other hand. Repeat these movements, grasping and stretching the muscles across the top of the shoulders.

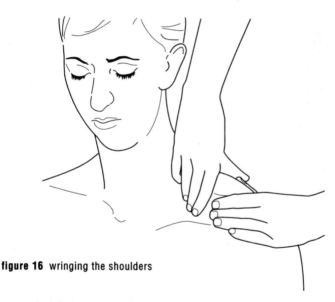

figure 16 wringing the shoulders

Benefits of petrissage

- increases blood supply bringing oxygen and nutrients to the area
- removes toxins from the deeper tissues
- breaks down tension nodules in the muscles
- relieves muscle spasm
- prevents stiffness after exercise

- breaks down fatty deposits
- aids relaxation
- stimulates the sebaceous glands.

Points to observe

- use the whole of the hand rather than just the fingers and thumbs which could cause pinching
- make sure that you are picking up the muscle rather than sliding your hands over the skin
- perform petrissage only on muscles and the more fleshy areas

Technique four – tapotement/percussion

Tapotement movements involve a series of light, brisk, springy actions applied with alternate hands in rapid succession. These movements are designed to stimulate and tone the treated area.

When performing tapotement your wrists need to be loose and flexible otherwise your movements may be too heavy and slow. The action comes from the wrists rather than the shoulders so you may find it useful to keep your elbows tucked in.

The main percussion movements used in Indian head massage include cupping, hacking, champi (double hacking), flicking and tapping (tabla playing). We will practise these movements individually.

1 Stand squarely behind your partner as before.
2 **Cupping.** Hold both hands above the receiver's shoulders and form a hollow curve with your fingers and thumbs. Bring your cupped hands down on to the top of the shoulders in quick succession. If you are performing the action correctly a hollow sound will be heard almost like a horse trotting. If it sounds like smacking then you need to cup your hands more!
3 **Hacking.** Hold your hands over the same area of the body with the palms facing each other, the thumbs uppermost. Flick your hands rhythmically up and down in rapid succession using the outer edge of your hands (the ulnar borders). Your movements should be light and springy and not like karate chopping!
4 **Champi (double hacking).** Place your hands together in a prayer position. Now allow them to relax so that the heels of the hands and the pads of the fingers and thumbs are gently touching. Perform light, rapid, striking movements with your fingers working across the shoulders briskly and rhythmically.

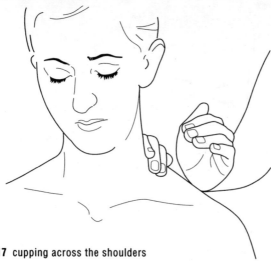

figure 17 cupping across the shoulders

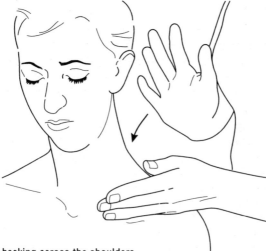

figure 18 hacking across the shoulders

5 **Flicking.** This is very similar to hacking and is often described as 'finger hacking'. To perform flicking bring *only* the sides of the little fingers into contact with the top of the shoulders rather than the edge of the hands. Once again work all the way across the shoulders.

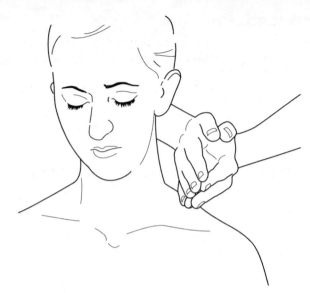

figure 19 champi

6 **Tapping/tabla playing.** *Tabla* refers to a drum used in the classical and popular music of northern India. It is such a light technique that it may be used on all areas of the body including the scalp, which is where we will practise it.

Hold both hands above the scalp and use your fingertips to gently tap all over the head. Try drumming using all your fingertips at once. Then try tabla playing using just one or two fingertips. Experiment with different rhythms – slow tapping is very soothing whereas rapid tapping is energizing and stimulating.

Benefits of tapotement
- stimulating and energizing
- improves the circulation to the area being treated
- increases muscle tone
- reduces fatty deposits
- when performed over the upper back it loosens mucus in the lungs.

Points to observe

- keep your wrists loose and movements light and springy
- when cupping ensure that your hands are cupped and not flat to avoid smacking
- when hacking do not tense up the fingers otherwise it could feel like karate chopping
- do not cup and hack on a sensitive area such as the face or the spine.

Technique five – chakra balancing

An Indian head massage is not complete until all the chakras have been balanced. Although the majority of therapists concentrate on just the three higher chakras, it is our opinion that it is essential to work on ALL the energy centres. Working on the three higher chakras only can make the receiver feel very light-headed, disorientated and ungrounded. An Indian head massage can leave one feel very 'spaced out' and it is essential to establish a sense of balance and a strong connection with the earth.

Chakra is a Sanskrit word which means 'wheel', 'disc' or ' circle'. The chakras are like constantly revolving wheels of energy which penetrate both the aura and the physical body. They can also be visualized as lotus flowers – each chakra having a different number of petals. The chakras act as a bridge between the physical body and the subtle bodies. There are seven major chakras which are described briefly here.

The base/root chakra

Sanskrit name: *Muladhara*.

Meaning: Root/support.

Location: Base of the spine in the perineum between the anus and genitals.

Colour: Red.

Element: Earth.

Function: Survival, grounding, security. It connects us with the physical world – the earth.

Glands connected with: Adrenals or some say gonads (i.e. testes/ovaries).

Crown Chakra

Third Eye/Brow Chakra

Throat Chakra

Heart Chakra

Solar Plexus Chakra

Abdomen/Sacral Chakra

Base/Root Chakra

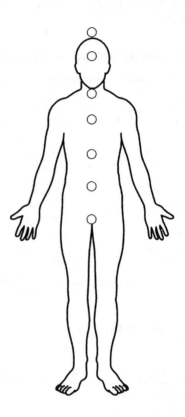

figure 20 chakras

Petals: Four.

Sound: LAM.

Physical imbalances include: The feet, ankles, knees, thighs, low back problems, sciatica, constipation and haemorrhoids. Lethargy (physical and mental) could result or an inability to sit still.

Psychological imbalances include: Feelings of 'spaciness', inability to ground oneself, insecurity.

The sacral/sexual/abdomen chakra

Sanskrit name: *Svadhisthana.*

Meaning: Seat of vital force/sweetness.

Location: Lower abdomen.

Colour: Orange.

Element: Water.

Function: Desire, sexuality.

Glands connected with: Ovaries/testes or some say spleen.

Petals: Six.

Sound: VAM.

Physical imbalances include: Malfunction of male/female sexual organs, impotence, frigidity, kidney or bladder problems, prostate problems and digestive problems.

Psychological imbalances include: Sexual perversion, promiscuity, possessiveness, greed.

The solar plexus/navel chakra

Sanskrit name: *Manipura.*

Meaning: Power chakra, lustrous gem.

Location: Between the navel and the solar plexus.

Colour: Yellow.

Element: Fire.

Function: Power.

Glands connected with: Pancreas or some say adrenals.

Petals: Ten.

Sound: RAM.

Physical imbalances include: Digestive problems such as stomach ulcers, diabetes, hypoglycaemia, allergies, anorexia, bulimia and chronic fatigue.

Psychological imbalances include: Low self-esteem, nervous exhaustion, addictions, mood swings, inability to relax.

The heart chakra

Sanskrit name: *Anahata*.

Meaning: Unstruck.

Location: Centre of chest.

Colour: Green (also pink).

Element: Air.

Function: Unconditional love.

Glands connected with: Thymus.

Petals: Twelve.

Sound: YAM.

Physical imbalances include: Asthma, blood pressure and circulatory problems, heart problems, respiratory disorders and poor immune system.

Psychological imbalances include: Depression, inability to love oneself and others, self-destructive, lack of compassion, inability to forgive.

The higher chakras

The throat chakra

Sanskrit name: *Visshuda*.

Meaning: Purification.

Location: Throat.

Colour: Blue.

Element: Sound/ether.

Function: Communication/creativity.

Glands connected with: Thyroid.

Petals: 16.

Sound: HAM.

Physical imbalances include: Throat problems, thyroid/para-thyroid problems, neck and shoulder problems, stuttering and non-stop verbal chatter.

Psychological imbalances include: Inability to express oneself, blocked creativity.

The third eye chakra

Sanskrit name: *Ajna*.

Meaning: To command, to know.

Location: Centre of forehead.

Colour: Indigo.

Element: Light.

Function: Intuition.

Glands connected with: Pituitary or some say pineal.

Petals: Two (the two physical eyes surrounding the third eye) or some say 96 (2 × 48).

Sound: OM.

Physical imbalances include: Eye/visual disorders, headaches, dizziness, nightmares.

Psychological imbalances include: Extreme confusion, halluci-nations, living in a fantasy world, lack of intuition.

The crown chakra

Sanskrit name: *Sahasrara*.

Meaning: Thousandfold.

Location: Crown of head (anterior fontanelle of a newborn baby).

Colour: Violet.

Element: Thought, knowing.

Functions: Understanding/bliss/enlightenment.

Glands connected with: Pineal or some say pituitary.

Petals: 1000.

Sound: Silent OM or silence.

Physical imbalances include: Epilepsy, Alzheimer's, Parkinson's disease, memory disorders.

Psychological imbalances include: Fear of opening up to spiritual levels, closed mind.

1 To balance the chakras position yourself behind the receiver with your weight evenly balanced, making sure that you feel a solid connection with the earth.
2 Place your hands very lightly on top of the receiver's shoulders or their head to establish an energy connection between the two of you.
3 Ask your partner to take a few deep breaths to release any tension and allow your breathing to synchronize with that of your partner.
4 Very gently lift your hands away from your partner's shoulders/head and move slowly to the side of the receiver. Place your hands just above the head and, without touching the physical body, try to tune into the chakras. You may feel sensations of heat or tingling or you may even see beautiful colours. With one hand at the front and one at the back, allowing them to hover a few centimetres away from your partner's body, move down the chakras.
5 Once you have reached the base chakra, move your hands slowly down the legs and place both hands on their feet. Rub their feet gently in order to ground them. Ask them to gently wriggle their fingers and toes and open their eyes when they are ready.
To ensure that they are completely earthed you may like to offer your massage partner a grounding stone such as black tourmaline, obsidian, smoky quartz or hematite.

Benefits of chakra balancing

• allows balance and harmony to be restored to body, mind and spirit
• releases energy blockages
• may prevent disease from occurring
• induces well-being, peace and love.

Points to observe

- make sure that you are properly earthed before beginning the chakra balance
- do not worry if you do not 'feel' anything at first – you may be trying too hard
- do not rush – take your time and allow both you and your massage partner to bathe in the peace and healing created by the balancing of the chakras
- ensure that the receiver is properly grounded at the end of the treatment and offer them a glass of water.

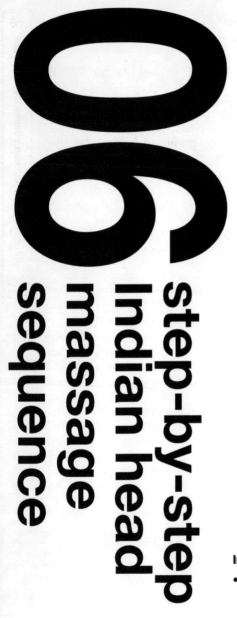

06

step-by-step Indian head massage sequence

In this chapter you will learn:

- how to carry out a complete Indian head massage treatment
- reactions to Indian head massage
- aftercare advice.

The easy to follow, step-by-step instructions and illustrations will enable you to carry out a complete Indian head massage simply, safely and effectively.

- **How long should an Indian head massage take?** A full treatment should take about 30 minutes. As you become more experienced it will take you even less time.
- **How many sessions will they need?** For maximum benefit, regular treatment is required. The ideal interval between Indian head massages is one week. This should keep your receiver calm and relaxed and far more able to cope with the pressures of life. The weekly interval between treatments allows time for self-healing to take place. If weekly sessions are not practical recommend an Indian head massage at least once a month.
- **How much pressure should I use?** The amount of pressure is determined by the individual you are working on and the area you are treating. The majority prefer a fairly firm pressure, but a more gentle touch is required for children or frail, delicate individuals. Far more pressure may be applied to the shoulders and upper back than the face. Adapt your treatment in accordance with the receiver's body language. Be aware of any signs of discomfort such as tensing or flinching – if this occurs, ease off the pressure. If your partner is showing signs of relaxation such as sighing and deep breathing, your touch must be just right. Simply use your common sense.
- **What reactions can I expect?** After an Indian head massage one or two reactions may occur. These reactions are a very positive sign and indicate that the body is clearing out mental and physical toxins and self-healing. Reactions will vary according to the individual. If someone has been under a great deal of stress and as a result has a considerable amount of muscular as well as nervous tension a reaction would not be unusual. This is a positive sign and shows that the body is coming back into balance.
  Reactions that may occur include:
  - a feeling of deep relaxation and tranquillity
  - relief from stress and tension
  - deeper and more refreshing sleep pattern
  - more clarity of thought
  - greater powers of concentration
  - increased alertness
  - tiredness due to the release of tension and toxins – followed by a feeling of revitalization

- aching and soreness in the muscles
- improved mobility in the neck and shoulders
- heightened emotional state as a result of balancing the chakras
- increased skin activity which may lead to pimples that quickly subside, resulting in a glowing complexion

It is a possibility that a mild reaction may emerge during the Indian head massage treatment. The receiver may become tearful as unwanted tension is released. Always be a good listener. Another very common reaction is a desire to fall asleep. This is to be encouraged so tell your massage partner not to fight sleep.

- **Posture.** Before you begin the importance of body posture needs to be emphasized. The correct use of posture while performing a treatment will increase the effectiveness of your treatment and prevent your back from discomfort.

Throughout the Indian head massage your back should be relaxed yet straight. Bend your knees slightly and tuck the bottom in so that your back can work from a secure base, namely, the pelvis. Your thighs should do most of the work not your back. Your feet should be placed firmly on the ground with your body weight evenly distributed – ensure that you are not leaning over to one side. Try to avoid looking down with your head forward all the time or your neck could ache. If you focus on your posture right from the beginning then you will not develop bad habits that are difficult to break. Remember it is as pleasurable to give an Indian head massage as it is to receive one.

Check!

- you have created a relaxing ambience for your massage (see pages 29–31)
- you have everything you will need for your treatment (see pages 31–32)
- you have taken note of any contraindications (see pages 37–40)
- you have prepared the receiver (see pages 35–36)
- you have prepared yourself properly (see pages 32–35).

Step-by-step sequence

N.B. If the receiver's hair is long, ensure that you tie or clip it up for the upper back, shoulders and neck sequence.

Connecting

Stand squarely behind the receiver. Lower your hands slowly and rest them very gently on the head. Ask the receiver to take a few deep breaths and allow your breathing to synchronize.

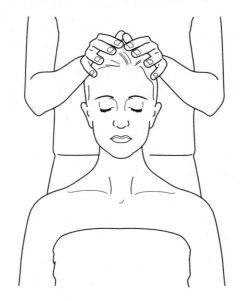

figure 21 connecting

Purpose
• helps to establish a bond
• allows you both to relax
• focuses your attention on the massage.

Upper back and shoulders

Benefits of Indian head massage

This is an area where most of us hold a great deal of tension. Driving a car, sitting at a computer or 'shouldering' responsibility are just a few factors that can make the upper back and shoulders stiff and inflexible. Indian head massage is excellent for releasing tension in this area.

1 Effleurage the upper back

Standing squarely behind the receiver place both hands, palms down, one on each side of the receiver's back, level with the bottom of the shoulder blades. Your fingers should be facing upwards.

Use the palmar surface of both hands simultaneously to stroke up the back and across the upper back and shoulders. Apply firm pressure on the upward stroke and glide back to your starting point with a feather-light touch. Commence using a light pressure gradually increasing the depth of your pressure. Repeat the effleurage movements until the muscles feel relaxed and warm.

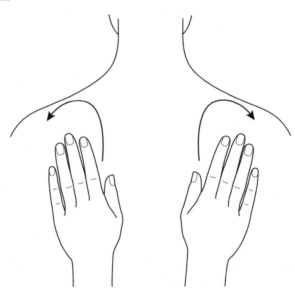

figure 22 effleurage

Purpose

- spreads the oil evenly (if used)
- familiarizes the receiver with your touch
- accustoms your hands to the receiver's body and allows you to determine the depth of pressure required
- improves circulation and lymph flow
- prepares the body for deeper movements.

2 Friction the upper back

Still standing behind the receiver, place the pads of the thumbs, one either side of the receiver's spine, level with the bottom of the shoulder blades.

Perform small, deep, circular outwards movements working up the back. As you reach the neck allow your hands to glide back to your starting position using no pressure. Repeat the friction several times trying to discover a 'knotty' area. When you encounter a nodule apply extra friction over the area gradually increasing the pressure. To achieve a deeper effect, place one thumb on top of the other and use your body weight to penetrate more deeply. Pressure should be firm yet not painful – be guided by your partner. If the friction becomes uncomfortable then ease off the pressure slightly.

Purpose
- breaks down knots and nodules
- improves circulation and lymph flow.

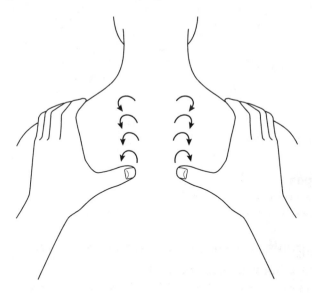

figure 23 friction on the back

3 Knuckle the upper back

Still standing behind your massage partner, make your hands into loose fists and place them on the back, level with the bottom of the shoulder blades.

Use both fists simultaneously circling in an outwards direction to knuckle up to the neck. Extra knuckling may be performed on troublesome areas.

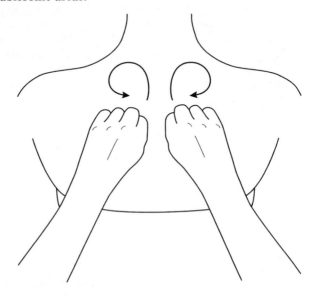

figure 24 knuckle the back

Purpose

• penetrates the tissues more deeply
• breaks down the fibrous adhesions even further.

4 Circular effleurage around the scapulae

Right scapula (shoulder blade)

Standing to the side of the receiver, place your left arm over the front of the receiver's shoulders and place your right hand on the right shoulder blade. Using the whole of your hand, make large circles around the entire shoulder blade. Repeat seven times, then effleurage the left shoulder blade.

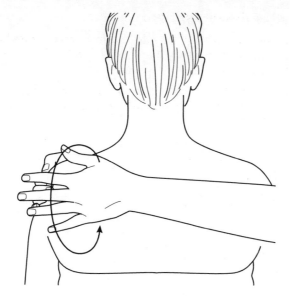

figure 25 circular effleurage around the scapula

Purpose
• prepares the shoulder blade for deeper movements.

5 Rubbing the scapula

Standing in the same position as for Step 4 place the whole of your hand, palm downwards, on the shoulder blade. Rub briskly and lightly across the top, middle and bottom of the shoulder blade. Repeat until you feel the warmth created by the rubbing under your hand. Repeat on the other scapula.

Purpose
• creates warmth in the area as the blood brings in oxygen and nutrients.

6 Friction the scapula

Standing in the same position as in Steps 4 and 5, place your thumb at the bottom of the scapula. Perform deep circular movements working all the way around the shoulder blade. If you encounter any knots use some extra friction to break them down. Friction may also be performed using the fingers instead of the thumbs. Repeat around the other scapula.

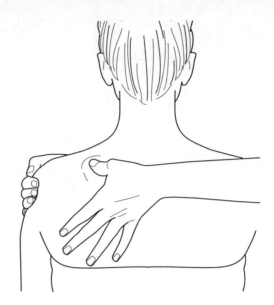

figure 26 friction the scapula

Purpose
- to break down knots and nodules
- to improve mobility of the scapula
- to provide pain relief.

7 Thumb pushes

Standing behind the receiver, place the palms of your hands at the corners of the shoulders with your thumbs at the back and your fingers resting at the front of the shoulders. Push your thumbs up and over the shoulder muscles. Repeat the thumb pushes in the middle of the shoulders and near the neck. Try to pick up as much muscle as you can as you push your thumbs over the shoulders. For a deeper movement try using the heels of your hands.

Purpose
- to loosen tension found across the shoulders
- to squeeze the toxins out of the shoulder muscles.

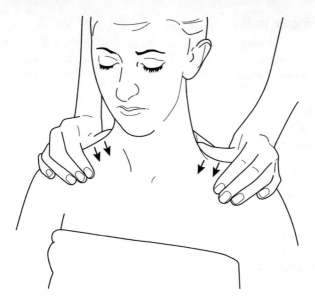

figure 27 thumb pushes on the shoulders

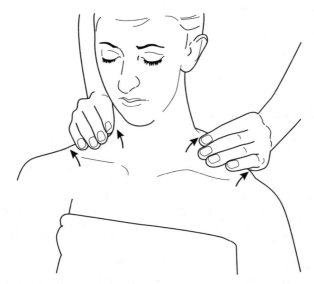

figure 28 finger pulls on the shoulders

8 Finger pulls

With your hands in the same position as in Step 7, use your fingers to pull back the muscles towards your thumbs. Perform this action several times and then repeat in the middle of the shoulders and near the neck.

Purpose
- to continue to loosen tight muscle fibres
- to squeeze the toxins to the surface.

9 Pick up and squeeze the shoulder muscles

Standing behind the receiver once again, place the palms of your hands onto the shoulders. Use the palms of your hands to pick up, squeeze and release the muscles. Always make sure that you are grasping and squeezing the muscles rather than the skin. It is the palms of your hands rather than your fingers that are doing most of the work.

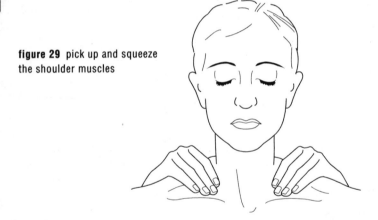

figure 29 pick up and squeeze the shoulder muscles

Purpose
- removes toxins from the deeper tissues
- breaks down tension nodules
- increases blood supply bringing fresh oxygen and nutrients.

10 Wring the shoulder muscles

Standing behind one shoulder, place the palms of both hands on top of the shoulder. Use one hand to pick up the muscle, squeeze it and pull it towards you. Then repeat the procedure using the

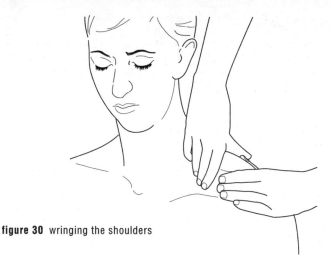

figure 30 wringing the shoulders

other hand. Repeat these movements rhythmically grasping and
stretching the muscles across the top of the shoulders.

Purpose

- loosens tight muscle fibres even further
- encourages the release of toxins from the deep tissues
- aids relaxation.

11 Tapotement across the shoulders

Cupping

Standing behind your partner form both hands into a hollow
curve. Bring your cupped hands down on to the shoulders in
quick succession. A hollow sound may be heard if you are
performing cupping correctly.

Hacking

Hold your hands, palms facing each other, thumbs uppermost
over the same area. Flick your hands rhythmically up and down
in rapid succession using the outer edge of your hands.

Champi (double hacking)

Place your hands together in a prayer position. Now allow them
to relax so that the heels of the hands and the pads of the fingers
and thumbs are gently touching. Perform light, rapid, striking
movements with the outer edge of your hands working across
the shoulders briskly and rapidly.

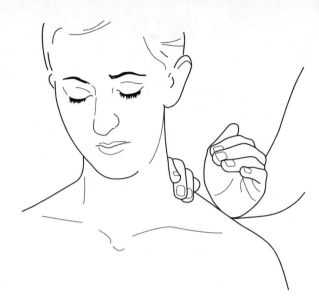

figure 31 cupping the shoulders

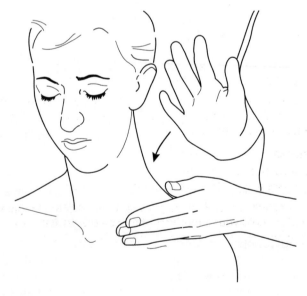

figure 32 hacking across the shoulders

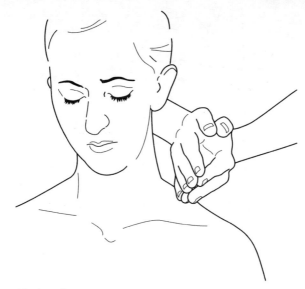

figure 33 champi

Purpose
- stimulates the circulation
- energizes and revitalizes
- improves poor muscle tone.

12 Smoothing across the shoulders

Standing behind the receiver, place one forearm on top of each shoulder. Apply medium pressure and glide across the top of the shoulders using your forearms.

Purpose
- drains away any toxins
- releases tension from the muscles.

To complete the step-by-step routine on the upper back and shoulders, hold your hands very gently on the receiver's shoulders. Notice how relaxed, warm and supple the shoulders feel.

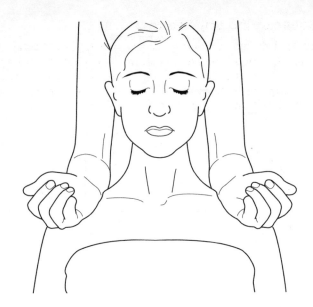

figure 34 smoothing across the shoulders

Arms

Benefits of Indian head massage

Our arms are in constant use as we go about our daily activities in the home, at work and in our leisure pursuits. Housework, carrying bags of shopping, walking the dog, working long hours at a computer or playing racket sports are just a few of the activities that put a strain on our arms.

1 Iron down the upper arms

Standing squarely behind your massage partner place both hands down, one on top of each shoulder. Stroke down from the top of the arms to the elbows using a firm pressure. Repeat this movement several times ensuring that you cover all aspects of the arms.

Purpose
- releases tension from the shoulders and upper arms
- helps to lower hunched-up shoulders
- drains toxins towards the lymph nodes in the axilla (armpit) and the elbow.

2 Squeeze the upper arms

Standing at the side of your massage partner, place the palms of your hands around the receiver's arm. One palm should be on the front of the upper arm and one on the back. Gently squeeze and release, working from the top of the upper arm down towards the elbow. Repeat on the other arm.

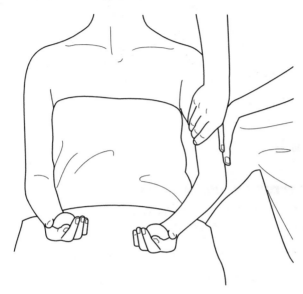

figure 35 squeeze the upper arms

Purpose
- encourages the deeper toxins to the surface
- releases toxins from the upper arms.

3 Squeeze and pick away

Still standing at the side of the receiver, clasp your hands, interlocking the fingers. Place your hands palms down on to the upper arm. Gently squeeze and lift away the muscles of the upper arm.

Purpose
- removes toxins from the deeper tissues
- loosens tight muscle fibres
- increases blood supply bringing fresh oxygen and nutrients.

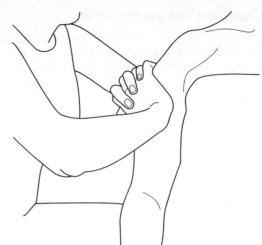

figure 36 squeeze and pick away

4 Heel roll the upper arms

Standing squarely behind the receiver, place your hands around the upper arms. Using firm pressure roll the heels of your hands over the muscles until they reach your fingertips. Repeat these movements in the middle of the upper arms and just above the elbows.

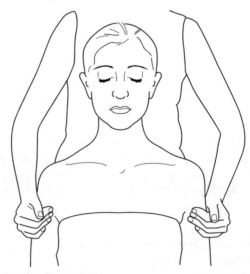

figure 37 heel roll the upper arms

Purpose

- loosens tension in the upper arms
- reduces aching and soreness
- creates warmth and increases lymph flow.

5 Shoulder mobilization

Standing to the side of the receiver, place one hand on the top of the shoulder and one hand under the elbow. Gently and slowly move the shoulder both clockwise and anticlockwise. Repeat on the other side.

Purpose

- improves mobility of the shoulder
- releases restrictions and tension around the shoulder joint.

6 Shoulder lift

Standing behind the receiver, place your hands just under their elbows. Ask them to take a deep breath and, as they inhale, keeping their arms close to the side, lift the arms upwards as far as is comfortable. As they breathe out allow the shoulders to return to their starting position. Repeat this lift three times.

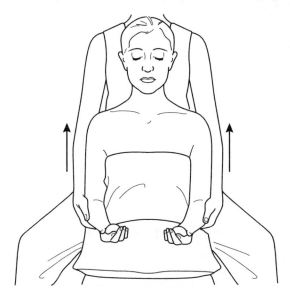

figure 38 shoulder lift

Purpose
- to release tension
- to drop the shoulders.

7 Iron the shoulders and upper arms

Standing behind the receiver, place both hands near the base of the neck. Stroke along the top of the shoulders and down the upper arms. Use fairly firm pressure to begin with and then a more gentle pressure to signal the end of the upper arm massage.

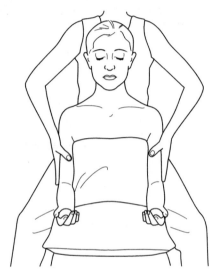

figure 39 iron the shoulders and upper arms

Purpose
- releases any remaining tension
- drains away toxins.

Neck

Benefits of Indian head massage

The neck area is extremely vulnerable to physical and emotional stress and tension. Contraction in the neck muscles is a major contributory factor to headaches. As well as tensing our neck muscles under stress, most of us will push our chins forwards as we go about our daily activities at work and in the home. The result is a permanently contracted state of the neck muscles leading to a considerable reduction in movement in the neck, tension headaches, migraines and eye strain.

Massage of the neck is an excellent way to relax tension in the neck and aid neck mobility. It can also help to improve posture.

1 Assess the tension in the neck

Standing to the side of the receiver, place one hand on the forehead and one hand at the back of the neck. Slowly and very gently rock your partner's head backwards and forwards three times.

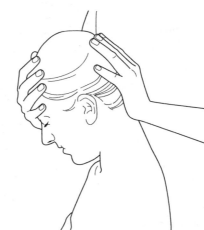

figure 40 assess the tension

Purpose
• enables you to assess how much tension there is in the neck

2 Effleurage the neck

Standing to the side of the receiver, place one hand on their forehead and ask him or her to drop the head slightly forwards so that you can support its weight. Use your other hand to stroke down the back and sides of the neck.

Purpose
• improves circulation, bringing warmth to the area
• encourages lymph flow
• releases tension
• prepares the neck for deeper movements.

3 Squeeze the neck

Still standing to the side of the receiver, place one hand on the forehead and this time ask your massage partner to tip their head backwards slightly. Place your working hand palm downwards on the back of the neck making a V-shape with your thumb and fingers. Gently and slowly squeeze and scoop up the muscles of the neck. Work the entire neck area from the base of the skull to the bottom of the neck.

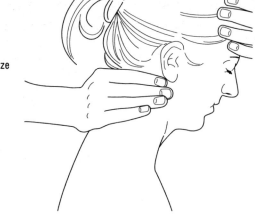

figure 41 squeeze the neck

Purpose
- loosens the neck muscles
- releases tension.

4 Friction the neck

Standing behind the receiver, tilt the head gently to one side. To support the head, place one hand on their forehead and cup your forearm around their head to allow it to rest comfortably and securely. Perform gentle circular friction movements with the pads of your fingers as you work down the back and one side of the neck. Now stand on the other side of your massage partner and repeat this technique.

Purpose
- breaks down knots and nodules
- brings increased circulation to the area.

5 Squeeze and release the side of the neck

Working in the same position as Step 4, form a V-shape with your thumb and fingers. Gently and slowly squeeze and release the muscles at the side of the neck. Repeat on the other side of the neck.

Purpose
- loosens the muscles at the side of the neck
- removes the toxins from the deeper tissues.

6 Thumb pushes to the side of the neck

Still working in the same position as for Steps 4 and 5, use your thumb to push the muscles forwards. Start just under the ear and perform thumb pushes right down the side of the neck. Repeat this technique on the other side of the neck.

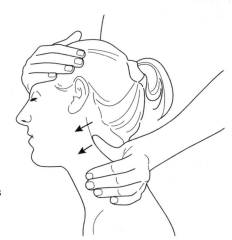

figure 42 thumb pushes to the side of the neck

Purpose
- helps to break down knots and nodules
- improves circulation and lymph flow.

7 Finger pulls to the side of the neck

Maintaining the same position as Steps 4–6, instead of pushing your thumbs forwards, draw the fingers back towards your thumbs. Work across the same area of the neck as before. Repeat on the other side of the neck.

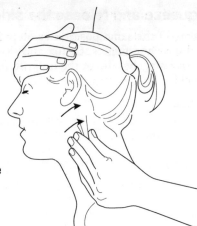

figure 43 finger pulls to the side of the neck

Purpose

- breaks down fibrous adhesions even further
- loosens the neck muscles.

8 Friction under the occiput (base of the skull)

Supporting the forehead with one hand use the pads of your fingertips to perform gentle circular friction movements all along the base of the skull.

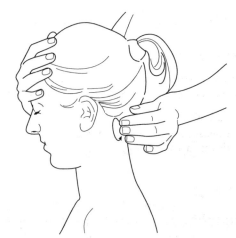

figure 44 friction under the skull

Purpose

- encourages tight muscles to release
- releases toxins and congestion from the base of the skull.

9 Heel rub under the occiput

Standing to the side of the receiver with one hand supporting the forehead, gently tilt the head forwards very slightly. Place the heel of your other hand at the base of the skull and perform light, brisk rubbing actions over the area.

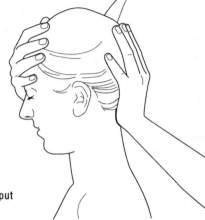

figure 45 heel rub under occiput

Purpose
- stimulates circulation encouraging a feeling of deep warmth
- encourages lymph flow
- relieves pain.

10 Completion

Standing to the side of the receiver to finish your massage of the neck, very gently stroke down the back and sides of the neck.

Purpose
- releases any remaining tension
- drains away toxins.

Scalp

Benefits of Indian head massage

It is incredible how tight the scalp can become as a result of tension. Such tightness in the scalp constricts the blood flow leading to headaches and poor-quality hair since the roots are starved of healthy nutrients. Indian head massage increases the circulation to the scalp, promoting hair growth. The hair becomes strong, shiny, healthy and lustrous. The sebaceous glands are stimulated, giving the hair a glossy appearance.

N.B. For the remainder of the step-by-step sequence, unclip the hair so that it is loose for best results. However, to make the movements clearer in the illustrations in this book the hair has been left clipped up.

1 Connect with the scalp

Standing squarely behind the receiver, gently rest your hands on either side of the receiver's head. As you connect try to become aware of how tense your partner's scalp is.

Purpose
• to assess the tension in the scalp.

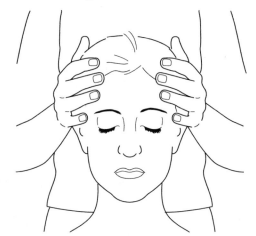

figure 46 connect with the scalp

2 Rub the side of the scalp

Standing slightly to the side of the receiver, place one hand on the side of the head for support. Use the heel of your working hand to perform light, brisk, rubbing movements starting from behind the ear and working in front of the ear and up towards the crown. Rub up and down the side of the scalp and then change hands to repeat this technique on the other side of the head. Now stand behind the receiver and use your whole hand to rub the top of the scalp. A zig-zag action is excellent.

Purpose

- stimulates the scalp
- increases circulation
- encourages activity of the sebaceous glands.

3 Friction with the whole hand

Standing behind the receiver, place both hands on top of the head. Use the whole of your hands to perform large circular friction movements over the entire scalp area. Pressure is fairly firm and eventually you should feel the scalp moving freely over the bone.

Purpose

- loosens up tight scalp muscles
- encourages circulation, sebaceous glands and lymph flow.

4 'Shampoo' the scalp

Still standing in the same position, place both hands on the receiver's head with your fingers well spread out in a claw-like position. Use the pads of your fingers and thumbs to perform small, slow, firm circular movements over the entire scalp. You should be able to feel the scalp moving beneath your fingers.

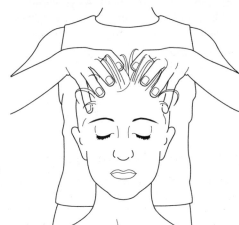

figure 47 shampoo the scalp

Purpose

- stimulates blood and lymph circulation
- loosens the scalp
- eases tension.

5 Ruffle the hair

Standing behind your massage partner, use the pads of the fingers and thumbs to gently ruffle the hair all over the scalp. Keep the wrists loose when performing this technique.

Purpose
- soothes the nerves
- encourages well-being.

6 Pluck the hair (soft landing, rapid take-off)

Standing behind the receiver make a loose claw shape with your hands and place the tips gently on the top of the head. Quickly lift your hands away bringing your fingers and thumbs together and 'land' in a different position. Repeat this technique all over the scalp.

Purpose
- stimulates hair growth
- energizes the receiver.

7 Tabla playing

Hold both hands above the scalp and use your fingertips to gently tap all over the head. As your fingers bounce off the scalp it is like raindrops falling. Drum using all your fingertips at once and then try tabla playing with just one or two fingertips.

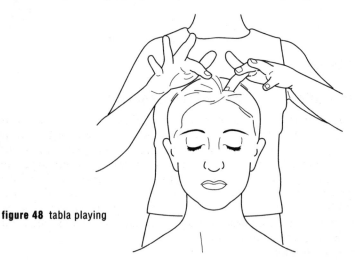

figure 48 tabla playing

Purpose
- energizes and stimulates
- induces well-being.

8 Stroke/comb through the hair

To complete the scalp sequence, stroke gently through the hair using the fingertips of both hands.

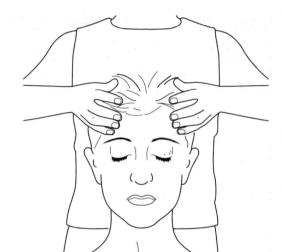

figure 49 stroke through the hair

Purpose
- encourages peace and tranquillity.

Face

Benefits of Indian head massage

Facial massage is wonderfully soothing and relaxing. It is immediately obvious just by looking at a person's face how uptight they are. The forehead frowns, the lips tighten and the jaw and teeth become clenched. As a result of facial massage you can look years younger without the need for botox and surgical procedures. As the circulation is improved, the complexion is rejuvenated and takes on a healthy glow. Even fine wrinkles can diminish or disappear. Massage of the face is also excellent for relieving sinus congestion.

N.B. It is important not to strain your partner's neck during the facial massage. Since the head needs to be tilted back very slightly, place a rolled-up towel or a small pillow behind the receiver's neck. Then allow their head to rest against your body.

1 Stroke the face

Standing behind the receiver, place the palms of your hands, fingers interlocking, on the receiver's forehead. Stroke outwards across the forehead. Let your hands glide back with no pressure.

To stroke the cheek area, place one hand on each cheek and stroke outwards towards the ears. Now stroke outwards across the chin and jaw. Repeat these techniques several times.

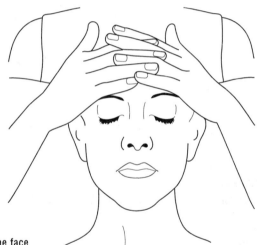

figure 50 stroke the face

Purpose
- relaxes the face muscles
- improves circulation and lymph flow.

2 Pressure points on the face

Standing behind the receiver, place the pads of both thumbs in the centre of the receiver's forehead just below the hairline. Slowly but firmly press and release, working outwards in a horizontal row. Work down the whole of the forehead in horizontal strips.

Repeat the same technique pressing and releasing in horizontal rows across the cheek area. The index finger may be used instead of the thumb. Now repeat the technique on the chin beginning just under the mouth working outwards in horizontal rows.

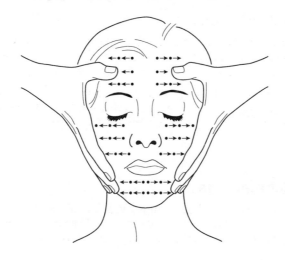

figure 51 pressure points – work in horizontal rows

Purpose
- pressure points help to clear sinuses
- encourages elimination of toxins
- improves blood flow to the area.

3 Circular temple friction

Standing behind your massage partner, place your hands on the temple area. Use the palms of the hands to make slow, circular movements. For a deeper movement, you may use the heels of the hands. For a lighter treatment, use the pads of the fingers.

Purpose
- relaxes and soothes
- relieves tension headaches
- relieves eye strain and relaxes the eyes.

figure 52 circular temple friction

4 Ear massage

Place the palms of your hands over the ears and perform very light outward circles over the ear area. Then gently squeeze and massage them between your thumbs and forefingers.

Purpose

• massaging the ears benefits all the systems of the body
• relaxes your massage partner.

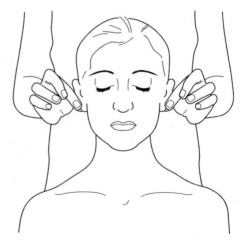

figure 53 ear massage

5 Massage around the eyes

Standing behind the receiver, use the pads of the index or middle fingers to very gently massage all around the eye sockets.

Purpose
- brings fresh blood to the eye areas
- clears congestion and puffiness
- makes the eyes look brighter and younger.

6 Release jaw tension

Standing behind the receiver, gently cup the jaw between your thumbs and index fingers. Very gently squeeze and release all along the jawline.

Purpose
- softens the jaw muscles
- releases tension and irritability.

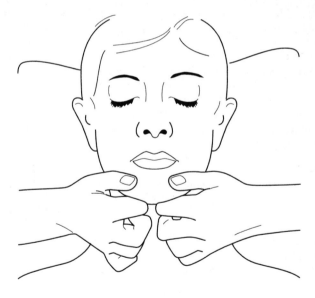

figure 54 release jaw tension

7 Facial tapping

Use the pads of your fingers to gently tap all over the face. It should feel like raindrops gently bouncing off.

Purpose
- stimulates the facial muscles
- improves circulation, inducing a healthy glowing complexion.

8 Final touch

Using your fingertips, gently stroke across the face using a feather-light touch.

Purpose
- completes the facial massage.

Chakra balancing

Standing at the side of the receiver, rest both hands very lightly on top of the receiver's head. Ask the receiver to take a few deep breaths and allow your breathing to synchronize. Lift your hands away and allow them to hover above your partner's head. With one hand at the back of the body and one hand at the front, glide them slowly down the body as you visualize the chakras. Now move to the front of your partner and glide down the legs and then place your hands on the feet. This will earth both you and your massage partner. If either of you feel 'spaced out', hold a grounding stone such as obsidian, black tourmaline, hematite or smoky quartz.

Purpose
- brings balance and harmony to body, mind and spirit
- releases energy blockages.

Aftercare advice

Immediately afterwards

Offer your partner a drink of water to assist the process of detoxification. They should be encouraged to sit quietly for a couple of minutes before rising. It is also a good idea to put on a warm jumper or sweatshirt. If you have used oil, advise the receiver to leave it on for a few hours after the treatment. This will allow the oil to penetrate, deeply nourishing hair, scalp and skin. When washing oily hair, a small amount of shampoo should always be applied straight onto the hair before wetting the hair.

In between treatments

The following aftercare advice will ensure that maximum benefits may be derived from the Indian head massage.

- **Increase intake of water.** Drinking water will assist the detoxification process. Water is the simplest, cheapest and most readily available way to improve our health. The World Health Organization recommends drinking eight glasses per day. However, research shows that just one in ten people drinks seven glasses or more daily.

  Therefore, the majority of us are chronically dehydrated and this puts a strain on the kidneys. This can give rise to infections such as cystitis and increases the likelihood of kidney stones. Dehydration can lead to other problems too, such as digestive and bowel problems (e.g. constipation) and headaches. Water increases the body's ability to fight off infections and greatly increases vitality. A 2 per cent drop in body water can trigger fuzzy short-term memory and difficulty in focusing on a printed page or computer screen. A large glass of water will also shut down hunger pangs. In fact, our thirst mechanism is so weak that we often mistake thirst for hunger. Water can even make us look younger. It plumps out the lines and gives the complexion a healthy, youthful glow.

- **Avoid eating heavy meals.** A heavy meal should definitely be avoided after a treatment, as a light diet is required while the body is using its energy for healing. A healthy diet can repair damage caused by years of eating abuse and should be regarded as an insurance policy. Fruits, vegetables and salads form a major part of a well-balanced diet. We should increase our fibre intake to reduce bowel problems. Refined carbohydrates, sugar, fat and salt should all be greatly reduced. Foods containing chemical additives and preservatives should be avoided altogether.

- **Reduce caffeine and alcohol intake.** Tea, coffee, cola and alcohol place an enormous strain on the body, particularly the kidneys. They also cause dehydration and headaches.

- **Avoid smoking.** Smoking, of course, is very dangerous to our health. It gives rise to all kinds of respiratory disorders and eventually often leads to cancer.

- **Take regular exercise.** The lifestyle of most of us, unfortunately, has become very sedentary. Instead of walking even small distances, the tendency is to take the car everywhere. Regular exercise increases energy levels and should become part of the daily routine. Try taking the stairs instead of the elevator and walking for a few minutes each day and you will notice the improvement. Exercise increases circulation and lymph flow, boosts the immune system, tones muscles, encourages deeper breathing and also releases toxins.

- **Get adequate sleep.** Sleep is vital for healing and is restorative. If we do not get enough sleep, we become grumpy and irritable and find the stresses and strains of everyday life much more difficult to cope with. The average sleep requirement is seven to eight hours per day. However, it does depend very much on the individual.

- **Take time to relax.** Try to ensure that you have time for rest and relaxation. Enjoy regular Indian head massage, pamper yourself with warm aromatherapy baths, listen to your favourite relaxation music and try some self-massage with essential oils.

- **Think positively.** Positive emotions such as love and laughter are important for reducing stress and boosting the immune system. A good laugh encourages happiness not only in yourself but also in those around you. It also speeds up the metabolic rate.

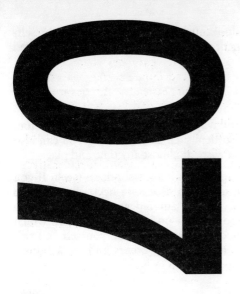

07

self-care

In this chapter you will learn:

- self-massage
- how to care for your hair
- how to promote a healthy, glowing complexion.

It is very important to look after your personal regime. A self-care routine should incorporate self-massage, hair care and looking after your skin.

Self-massage

Self-massage is a wonderful way to soothe away stress and tension, and to treat common disorders such as headaches. You can also perform it as often as you wish, at almost any time and place.

Ideally you should massage yourself at least once a week. If you are experiencing discomfort such as a sore neck, massage the affected area daily. You will be amazed at the relief. As you perform the massage movements on yourself, discover which ones feel particularly good. As you practise on yourself you will become more proficient at massaging others and, as a bonus, your health will improve.

Neck and shoulders

Tightness in the neck and shoulders is an extremely common symptom of stress and often gives rise to headaches. These simple techniques can help to break down the numerous knots and nodules which arise and will improve neck mobility enormously. Try these movements when you feel stressed or to prevent headaches from occurring.

Position for massage: Sitting on a chair, bed or the floor.

1 Neck – effleurage
Relax your neck forwards and place your hands behind your head, fingertips touching or slightly overlapping. Apply deep, effleurage movements across and down the neck.

2 Neck – friction
Apply small circular friction movements to the base of your skull using your fingertips.

3 Shoulders – effleurage
Place one hand on each shoulder near the base of the neck. Stroke both hands across your shoulders. For a deeper treatment to massage your right shoulder, reach across the front of your chest and place your left hand at the base of the skull and stroke firmly down the side of the neck and over your shoulder. Repeat on the other shoulder.

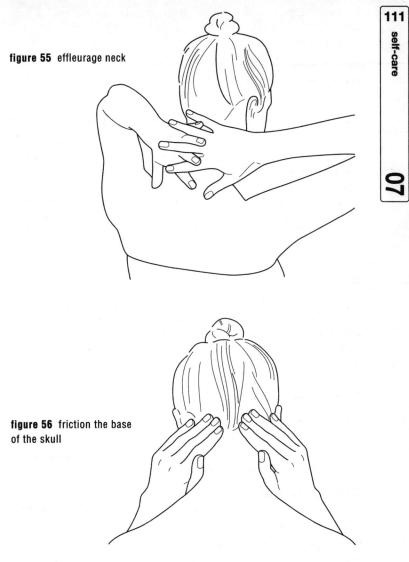

figure 55 effleurage neck

figure 56 friction the base of the skull

4 Shoulders – pick up and squeeze

Reach across the front of your chest again and squeeze and release the muscles on top of the other shoulder, picking up as much flesh as possible. Repeat Steps 3 and 4 on the other shoulder.

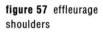
figure 57 effleurage shoulders

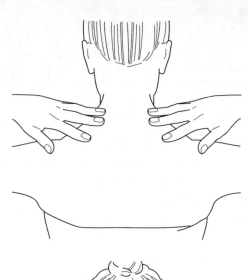

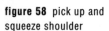
figure 58 pick up and squeeze shoulder

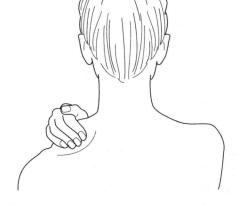

5 Scapulae – friction

Reach across the front of your body with your right hand to touch your left shoulder blade at the back of your body. Use your fingertips to apply deep pressure to any knots or nodules. Repeat on the other scapula.

Arm and hand

Our arms, wrists and hands are used constantly in our daily activities. Aches and pains in the arms and hands are often caused by repetitive movements, although they may be the result of a neck problem. Massage of these areas is essential to promote strength and mobility and is particularly beneficial to people who use their hands and arms extensively in the course of their work, for example, individuals who use computer keyboards and gardeners and hairdressers. Treatment is also essential for sports people for preventing injuries. According to hand reflexology, all the parts of the body are mirrored in miniature on the hands. For further information please refer to *Teach Yourself Hand Reflexology*.

Position for massage: Sitting down on the floor, bed or a chair. Rest your hands gently on your lap.

1 Arm – effleurage
Place the palm of your hand on your wrist and effleurage the whole of the arm up to the shoulder.

2 Upper arm – effleurage
Apply deep stroking to the flexor muscles on the front of your upper arm and the extensor muscles on the back of your upper arm. Always work up your arm trying to move the lymph up the axillary glands in your armpit.

3 Upper arm – petrissage
Squeeze and wring the muscles of your upper arm to break down any adhesions and to bring the deeper toxins to the surface.

4 Lower arm – deep stroking
With your elbow flexed and the tip of your elbow resting on your abdomen to encourage drainage, apply deep downward longitudinal stroking to the flexor and extensor muscles on the front and back of your lower arm.

5 Wrist – loosen and move
Use your thumb and fingertips to gently friction all around the wrist joint. After these loosening movements, interlock your fingers and circle the wrist clockwise and anticlockwise.

6 Palm – circular kneading
With a clenched fist, work into the palm of your hand with circular movements to loosen up the muscles, tendons and joints.

7 Fingers and thumb – loosen and move
Using your thumb and index finger gently stretch each finger and thumb. Then circle each one individually. These movements will ease rheumatic complaints and arthritis.

Face and scalp

Face and scalp massage is a wonderful way to relax and unwind, completely banishing tiredness and anxiety, relieving headaches and clearing sinuses. Over a period of time, as circulation and drainage is stimulated, you will also notice improvements in your complexion and fine wrinkles may disappear.

Position for massage: Lying down on the floor or bed or sitting up on a chair if you prefer.

1 Face effleurage
Place both hands palms down on your forehead with your fingertips facing each other. Stroke across your forehead. Repeat this outward movement stroking across your cheeks and across your chin.

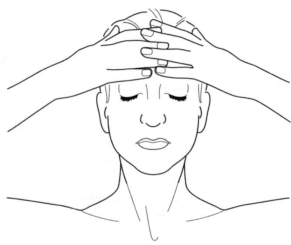

figure 59 stroke the face

2 Eyes – stroking
Use your index or your index and middle fingers to very gently effleurage outwards underneath each eye. Take great care, as this is a very delicate area. These movements will help to relieve puffiness and to prevent and reduce fine lines.

3 Chin and jaw – toning
Pinch all along your jawline using your thumbs, index and middle fingers to help prevent a double chin.

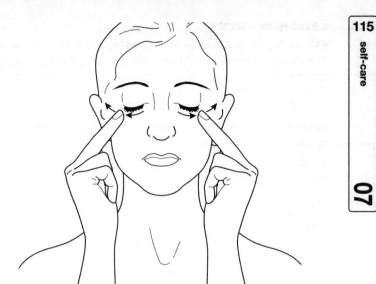

figure 60 stroke gently under each eye

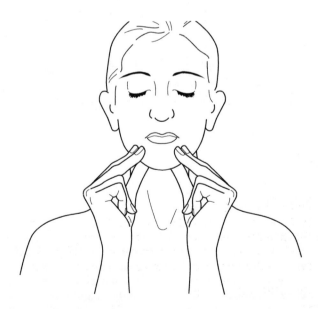

figure 61 tone the chin and jaw

4 Eyebrows – toning

Starting at the inside of your eyebrows, pinch your brow bone until you reach the end of your eyebrow. Repeat each movement several times.

5 Mouth – friction

Make a large 'O' with your mouth. Using your index and middle fingers apply small circular friction movements around your mouth. These movements may help to stop fine wrinkles appearing.

6 Scalp – friction

With your fingertips, use small rotary movements covering your entire scalp. These movements will remove tension from your scalp and, by aiding circulation, can also make your hair healthier.

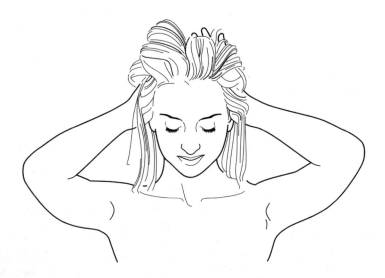

figure 62 scalp friction

7 Completion

To finish your massage programme, place the heels of your hands over your eyes. Hold your hands there for a few seconds allowing your eyes to relax completely in darkness; as you gently remove your hands you will feel revitalized and refreshed.

Hair care

Our hair is a reflection of our inner health. The condition of the hair is dependent on many factors – nutrition, hormonal changes, hereditary factors, stress, overexposure to sun, chemicals such as from perms, dyes and hairsprays, and pollutants and drugs. Correct washing of the hair and regular scalp massage using oils and essential oils can help to keep your hair strong, shiny and lustrous.

Washing your hair

Most commercial shampoos contain chemical and synthetic substances that damage the scalp and hair follicles. They attack the acid mantle and rid the hair of its natural protective oils. After each washing we recommend that you rinse your hair with an acidic substance such as lemon juice or organic cider vinegar. This will wash out any residues of soap and help to restore the acid equilibrium of the scalp. Avoid using the harsh, detergent-based shampoos. Instead choose a mild, natural shampoo or try making your own using the following recipe:

100 g soap flakes
1 l spring water

Simmer the spring water and add the soap flakes until the flakes dissolve. Allow the mixture to cool and store in a bottle or jar. Either 100 ml or 250 ml HDP (high-density polythene) bottles are ideal for this purpose and are available from reputable suppliers (see 'Useful addresses' page 128).

You may add carrier oils and essential oils to this shampoo, depending upon your hair type. Here, for the sake of simplicity we will only use the top ten essential oils outlined in Chapter 04: bergamot, carrot seed, chamomile, frankincense, geranium, lavender, lemon, rose, rosemary and tea tree.

Normal hair

Normal hair is neither dry nor greasy. It is strong, shiny and easy to comb. Here are some tips for maintaining your healthy head of hair.

Essential oils for normal hair
- carrot seed
- chamomile

- geranium
- lavender
- lemon
- rosemary.

Choose any of these oils and add them to your natural shampoo base. Chamomile and lemon are excellent for fair hair, rosemary will enhance dark hair and carrot seed is beneficial for ginger hair.

Blond hair

Eight drops chamomile
Eight drops lemon } added to 100 ml shampoo base
Eight drops geranium

Dark hair

Eight drops carrot seed
Eight drops lemon } added to 100 ml shampoo base
Eight drops rosemary

At least once a week, massage your hair with nourishing hair oil. This is particularly important if hair is washed frequently, exposed to the sun, wind or chlorine and, if this is the case, it is necessary to massage the scalp at least twice a week. A treatment using one of the following blends will condition your hair.

Blond hair

Two drops chamomile
Two drops geranium } blended with 10 ml of carrier oil

Dark hair

One drop geranium
One drop lemon } blended with 10 ml of carrier oil
Two drops rosemary

Massage the oil thoroughly into the hair and scalp, and then cover the head with a plastic shower cap. The oil should be left on the hair for at least an hour and, if possible, overnight.

Dry hair

Dry hair is due to inactivity of the sebaceous glands. Head massage is an excellent way to stimulate them.

Essential oils for dry hair

- carrot seed
- chamomile
- geranium
- lavender.

Any of these oils may be added singly or in a combination to your shampoo base. We recommend:

Eight drops chamomile
Eight drops geranium   } added to 100 ml shampoo base
Eight drops lavender

Dry hair which has been damaged by bleach and the sun needs a considerable amount of nourishment and care. The following recipe is recommended for use twice a week. You could make up a large batch, store it in an amber glass bottle to prevent it from damage and then, in between treatments, massage a small amount into any dry areas such as the ends of your hair.

One drop carrot seed
Two drops geranium   } blended with 10 ml of carrier oil
One drop lavender

Oily hair

Oily hair is caused by an overactivity of the sebaceous glands. This condition is exacerbated by shampooing too often with commercial shampoos.

Essential oils for oily hair

- bergamot
- frankincense
- lavender
- lemon
- rosemary.

Add any of these oils to your shampoo base. An effective blend is:

Eight drops bergamot
Eight drops frankincense } added to 100 ml shampoo base
Eight drops lemon

Oily hair will benefit from a hair tonic which should be rubbed into the scalp and, if possible, left overnight:

Two cups spring/boiled water

Two tablespoons fresh lemon juice

Two drops bergamot

Two drops frankincense

Two drops lavender

Blend well and rub into an oily scalp.

You may think that because your hair is oily it is not necessary to massage your scalp with oil. On the contrary, oily hair needs conditioning too. Try the following recipe:

One drop bergamot
One drop frankincense } blended with 10 ml of carrier oil
One drop lavender
One drop rosemary

Other hair tips

- use a wide-toothed comb for wet hair because it is very fragile and can easily be damaged
- try to allow your hair to dry naturally yet away from direct sunlight
- minimize blow-drying. if you must blow-dry your hair, set the hair dryer on medium heat and hold it at a sensible distance, about 20 cm away from your hair
- minimize the use of curling tongs, heated rollers and crimpers etc.
- avoid chemical processes such as perming and colourings
- protect your hair from sunlight, sea and chlorinated swimming pools
- eat a healthy diet
- relax as much as possible since stress can make you lose your hair.

Skin care

Our skin is also a reflection of our inner health. Commercially produced cosmetics contain a whole host of synthetic substances such as preservatives, dyes and fragrances. These damage the skin's flora and protective 'acid mantle' and promote ageing of the skin. Indian head massage is an excellent way of improving your complexion, making it smooth and silky. The oils will encourage the shedding of old skin cells and the regeneration of new ones. The sebaceous glands will function more efficiently and the pores will be cleansed thoroughly, flushing out the toxins. All in all a healthy, flawless, soft, fresh, glowing complexion is promoted. Massage your face daily as directed on pages 114–116 and you will notice a difference.

Normal skin

Normal skin is smooth, fine pored, soft and supple with no blemishes. Such a flawless complexion is often found in children whereas the rest of us have to work hard to achieve it! However, there will be times when normal skin becomes unbalanced due to hormonal problems, illness or a change in diet.

Essential oils for normal skin
- chamomile
- frankincense
- geranium
- lavender
- rose.

Select any one of the essential oils or a combination from the list above and add them to a carrier oil. Base oils particularly recommended for normal skin include apricot kernel, jojoba, peach kernel and sweet almond oil. Mix up your own special aromatherapy facial oil and store in an amber-coloured glass bottle. Massage the oil into your face once a day as directed in the self-massage section.

One drop chamomile

Two drops geranium

One drop lavender

} blended with
10 ml
of carrier oil

Normal skin will benefit from the occasional facial steam bath. This will cleanse the pores thoroughly, flush out the toxins and stimulate the circulation. To prepare a facial steam bath, boil

500 ml–1 l of water and pour into a bowl. Add six drops of your chosen essential oil. Bend your head over the bowl, cover your head with a towel and steam your face for approximately ten minutes.

Dry skin

The lack of moisture in dry skin is due to inactive sebaceous glands which are not producing sufficient sebum. Dry skin is prone to more wrinkles than any other skin type and needs to be fed daily with nourishing and protective oils.

Essential oils for dry skin

- carrot seed
- chamomile
- frankincense
- geranium
- lavender
- rose.

Any of these essential oils may be added to a nourishing carrier oil such as apricot kernel, borage seed oil, evening primrose oil, jojoba, peach kernel or sweet almond. Avocado is penetrating but rather thick and sticky to use on its own – only add a small amount to your main carrier oil.

One drop carrot seed

One drop frankincense } blended with 100 ml of carrier oil

One drop rose

If you have dry skin, it is advisable to avoid hot facial steam baths and hot facial masks. Instead, try a lukewarm facial compress. To prepare a compress, heat up approximately 25 ml of water and pour into a bowl. Add four drops of your chosen essential oil and stir. Dip a face flannel into the bowl and place it on your forehead until it cools off. Repeat the procedure on your cheeks and chin.

Oily skin

Oily skin is a result of an overactivity of the sebaceous glands. It is most common during puberty due to the hormonal changes that are taking place. The pores of the skin become clogged and tend to form spots, blackheads and even acne. Problem areas particularly affected include the nose, chin, cheeks and forehead.

Essential oils for oily skin

- bergamot
- frankincense
- geranium
- lavender
- lemon
- rosemary.

Select any of the essential oils from the list above and add them to a favourite carrier oil such as apricot kernel, calendula oil, peach kernel or sweet almond. Massage your blended aromatherapy oil into the face daily.

One drop bergamot

One drop frankincense $\left.\right\}$ blended with 10 ml of carrier oil

One drop lemon

If you have individual spots or blackheads, these may be treated individually with one drop of neat lavender or tea tree applied with a cotton bud. Do take care around the eye area.

Oily skin will benefit from a facial steam bath to eliminate the toxins and thoroughly cleanse the pores. Follow the directions on pages 121–122 in the section on normal skin.

Face masks are a must for oily skin to cleanse, tone and invigorate. The most important ingredient of a face pack is Fuller's earth or clay which will draw the toxins out. A face mask should be given once a week.

Face mask for oily skin

Two tablespoons of clay/Fuller's earth

One teaspoon lemon pulp

One teaspoon water

One teaspoon honey

One drop geranium

One drop lemon

All the above ingredients should be mixed together to form a paste. This should be applied to the face, avoiding the eye area, and left on until it is dry. Carefully wash it off using a warm, damp flannel.

Other skin tips

- pay attention to your diet. include lots of fresh fruit, vegetables and salad and drink at least eight glasses of water daily
- do not smoke or drink large amounts of alcohol, tea, coffee or drinks containing caffeine since these give rise to prematurely aged skin
- take regular exercise to increase the circulation
- try to avoid extremes of temperature such as strong sunlight and wind
- avoid stress since it is very ageing
- if you have problem skin, supplements of zinc, evening primrose oil and vitamin C can be helpful
- avoid using synthetic cosmetics since these may promote ageing of the skin.

I hope that you have enjoyed practising the wonderful therapy of Indian head massage on your family and friends. If you have been inspired by this book and have received positive feedback, you may decide that you wish to take a professional Indian head massage course. There are many short courses available at colleges of further education, which will give you the skills to develop your hobby. If you would like to become professionally qualified, however, it is important to seek out a reputable establishment (see 'Useful addresses', page 128). A recognized course will involve a study of anatomy and physiology. At the end of the course you will be required to take both theory and practical examinations and, in addition, you will be expected to carry out case studies.

Tips for choosing a course

- study several different prospectuses before making your choice
- make an appointment to view the college preferably on a day when an Indian head massage course is running; stay for tea break to speak with the current students who will be able to give you a good impression of what the college is really like
- meet the tutor. How long has he/she been practising? Do they still run a practice? What are their qualifications? Do they hold a recognized teaching qualification?
- how long has the college been established?
- what is the examination pass rate?
- is the school accredited to a reputable association?
- will you be able to gain insurance to practise after completion of the course?

- do they have former students you can talk to about the course?
- ask to see some of the former students' work and some case histories.

Do not part with any fees until you are completely satisfied with the college. By far the best way to choose an Indian head massage course is recommendation.

The future

Indian head massage is dramatically increasing in popularity as a therapy. It is practised in health clinics, on health farms, in private practices, on airplanes, in offices, at conferences, in beauty clinics, hairdressing salons, rehabilitation centres, cruise liners and so on. Therapists either practise Indian head massage in its own right or they combine it with complementary therapies such as massage, aromatherapy or reflexology. Whether you decide to practise Indian head massage professionally or as a hobby, the choice is yours! I do hope that it will become part of your daily routine.

further reading

The author, Denise Whichello Brown, is an international authority on complementary therapies. If you have enjoyed this book why not read her other books in this series:

Teach Yourself Aromatherapy

Teach Yourself Hand Reflexology

Teach Yourself Massage

useful addresses

Beaumont College of Natural Medicine

MWB Business Exchange, Hinton Road, Bournemouth BH1 2EF. Tel: +44 (0)1202 708887. Fax: +44 (0)1202 708720. http://www.beaumontcollege.co.uk

Information on training courses under the direction of Denise Brown.

Denise Brown Essential Oils

MWB Business Exchange, Hinton Road, Bournemouth BH1 2EF. Tel: +44 (0)1202 708887. Fax: +44 (0)1202 708720. http://www.denisebrown.co.uk

A wide selection of high-quality, pure, unadulterated essential oils, base oils, creams and lotions, relaxation music etc. is available from Denise Brown Essential Oils (International Mail Order).

glossary

acne Acne occurs primarily during puberty but it can affect people well into their adult years. It is due to overactivity of the sebaceous (oil secreting) glands of the skin. Excessive sebum causes proliferation of bacteria, and the pores become blocked leading to blackheads and spots. It can lead to scarring.

alopecia Loss or absence of hair usually noticeable on the scalp which is often hereditary but may be due to stress.

anaemia Common blood disease characterised by a deficiency of the haemoglobin (iron containing) component of the red blood cells. Symptoms include fatigue, shortness of breath, dizziness, fainting, pallor of the skin and disturbed appetite.

antibacterial Destroys or hinders the growth of bacteria.

antiviral Inhibits the proliferation of viruses.

antifungal Destroys or prevents the growth of fungi.

antidepressant Helps to prevent depression.

antiparasitic Destroys parasites such as lice.

aromatherapy The use of essential oils to balance body, mind and spirit.

atlas First vertebra in the neck.

axis Second cervical vertebra.

Ayurveda An ancient system of medicine that has been practised in India for thousands of years. It is a Sanskrit word derived from two roots 'ayur' which means 'life' and 'veda' meaning 'knowledge' or 'science'. Ayurveda stresses the holistic principle to bring the body back to a state of equilibrium and prevent disease from occurring.

adhesions Muscle fibres that adhere together to form a hard lump or knot.

arthritis   Osteoarthritis is a common degenerative disorder that mostly affects the weight bearing joints such as the hips and knees.

base/carrier/fixed oil   A vegetable oil such as sweet almond in which essential oils are diluted for massage.

chakra   A Sanskrit word meaning 'wheel', 'disc' or 'circle'. The chakras are also known as energy centres. There are seven major chakras.

champi (otherwise known as double hacking)   A technique that energizes and revitalizes.

circulatory system   Consists of the heart, arteries, veins, capillaries and the blood.

conjunctivitis   An inflammation of the lining of the eyelid where the eye becomes red, swollen and discharges. It is easily spread from one eye to the other.

cupping   A massage technique performed by bringing cupped hands in quick succession down on to a fleshy area that makes a hollow sound if performed correctly.

dandruff   A common condition whereby dead skin is shed excessively from the scalp producing white flakes in the hair.

dermatitis   Inflammation of the skin that may be due to an allergy or an unknown cause.

eczema   Inflammation of the skin characterized by scaling or blisters.

effleurage   A stroking movement that if performed slowly has a calming and soothing effect on body and mind. Brisk effleurage energizes, revitalizes and banishes tiredness.

endorphins   'Happy hormones' that produce a sense of elation and well-being and relieve pain.

essential oil   The odiferous, volatile component of an aromatic plant.

frictions   Deep penetrating movements useful for locating and breaking down knots and nodules.

hacking   A massage technique whereby the outer edges of the hands are flicked up and down in rapid succession.

head lice   The head louse is a small parasite that feeds on blood from the scalp. Nits are found in the hair close to the scalp and the person will complain of itching. The scalp may look red due to itching.

haemorrhage   Excessive bleeding.

herpes simplex This virus is present in approximately 90 per cent of the population and may be activated by stress, ill health or sunlight. It is commonly found around the lips and begins as an itching sensation followed by the appearance of small blisters around the mouth. These weep and form crusts and persist for approximately two to three weeks.

hypertension High blood pressure.

hypotension Low blood pressure.

impetigo A highly infectious and contagious disease caused by streptococcal and staphylococcal bacteria. It is most commonly found on the face near the mouth, nose and around the ears but it may appear on the scalp. It is indicated by blisters usually in groups, which burst and then dry leading to the formation of yellow crusts.

insomnia Difficulty in sleeping. As many as one in three adults suffer from it at some time in their lives.

lymphatic system Helps to drain away excess tissue fluid, harmful wastes and toxins and plays a vital role in the body's defence and immune system.

migraine A severe headache usually one sided and can be accompanied by nausea, vomiting and visual disturbances.

myalgic encephalomyelitis (M.E.) A disorder characterized by severe muscle fatigue, weakness and exhaustion. It is also known as post-viral fatigue syndrome.

osteoporosis A condition most common after the menopause characterized by brittle bones that are more easily fractured.

parkinson's disease A disease of the nervous system causing muscle tremor, stiffness and a shuffling walk.

petrissage A massage technique meaning to knead whereby the soft tissues are picked up and lifted from the underlying structures, compressed and then released.

psoriasis This condition is characterized by the formation of red patches which are covered by scaly skin, occurring mostly on the elbows, knees, palms of the hands, soles of the feet and on the head. Psoriasis is often inherited but may not appear until adulthood. The cause is unknown, although stress appears to be a major factor.

scabies A skin infestation caused by a mite which burrows into the skin and lays eggs. It is highly contagious.

sebaceous glands Secrete sebum which keeps the skin moist and gives the hair a glossy sheen.

sinusitis A painful inflammation of the membrane lining the facial sinuses caused by infection. It may develop as a complication of the common cold. Symptoms include a throbbing ache and a feeling of fullness and the sufferer may lose his/her sense of smell.

stye A small pus-filled abscess near the eyelashes caused by an infection.

tabla playing A light technique performed by gently tapping the fingertips. A 'tabla' is a drum used in the music of northern India.

tapotement/percussion Light, brisk springy movements applied with alternate hands in rapid succession designed to stimulate and tone an area.

tinea capitis Tinea capitis is a fungal infection that appears as round circular patches that may look red and scaly and can itch. (Tinea corporis is ringworm of the body).

tonic Strengthens and enlivens the whole body.